# Simple Moves

## For

## The

## Body & Soul

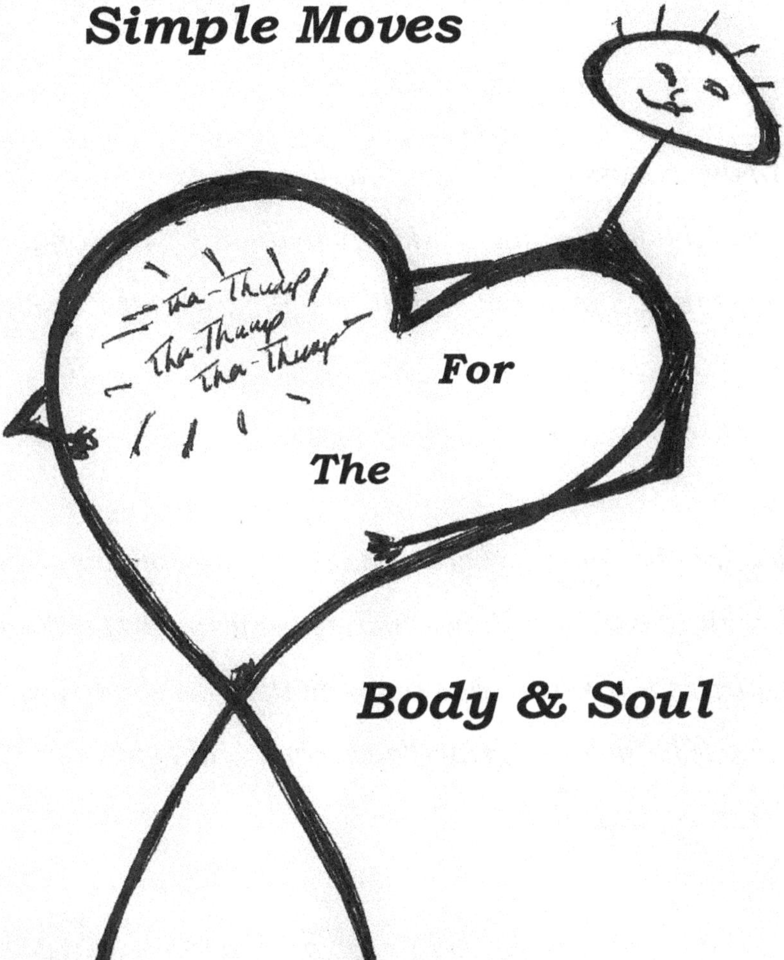

*A Whole ~ Body Wellness Guide*

# Jana Lee

## *Simple Moves For The Body & Soul*

*An awareness of abilities and disabilities of being home bound is the inspiration to share the author's personal and wellness fitness programs. Follow along, with the stories; recipes; laughter and tears. Humor is essential to the body's healing.*

*To find that place where mind and body connect we must realize their purpose. As we increase our understanding, our spirit is awakened, and our soul delights. Including the whole self helps us to grow; learn; and build stronger, healthier relationships.*

*Use caution and care: For the body as well as the soul; that your life may be enriched through this journey along a path to health.*

Published by:
Dove Tail Publishing
PO Box 1353
Shady Cove, Oregon 97539

Cell Phone: 1-425-418-1009

Manufactured in:

The United States of America

ISBN: 978-0-578-00982-7

**2009 Copyrights: Jana Lee**
All rights reserved. Permission must be obtained, in writing, from the author, prior to copying any portion of this book, for any reason, including storage and retrieval, by photographic, mechanical, electronic or any other method.
Contact the author: Jana Lee
By Telephone: 1-425-418-1009
By E-Mail: janaleebooks@gmail.com

*Dedicated*
*To all those*
*With limited abilities*
*Physical; Emotional; and Spiritual*

*Simple Moves For The Body & Soul*

# Where to Find:
## *Chapter ~ Topic ~ Page*

One:       The Connection of Body, Mind & Heart     15

Two:       Let's Talk About Health     23

Three:     Things We Should Do     31

Four:      The Food We Eat     39

Five:      A to Z List of Feel ~Good Foods     49

Six:       Healthy Recipes & Creative Cooking     57

Seven:     A Few Quick & Easy Ideas     67

Eight:     Environments We Live and Work In     73

Nine:      Emotional Roller Coasters     79

Ten:       Aware of the Body's Abilities     87

Eleven:    Family and Social Life     95

Twelve:    Respect: in Layman's Terms     103

Thirteen:  Let's Talk About Fitness     111

Fourteen:  Recipes: Quick & Easy Starts & Snacks     117

*Simple Moves For The Body & Soul*

# *Where to Find:*
## *Chapter ~ Topic ~ Page*

Fifteen:     Let's Talk a Little More About Faith     129

Sixteen:     Endurance     135

Seventeen:     Building a Positive Well Being     141

Eighteen:     And, About Life     149

Nineteen:     Humans Really Are Insecure Creatures     157

Twenty:     About Our Foods     167

Twenty One:     How Food Counts     175

Twenty Two:     Add a Little Laughter     183

Twenty Three:     About Exercise     191

Twenty Four:     Life Changes ~ For the Soul     207

Twenty Five:     Relationship ABC's     215

Twenty Six:     Whole Body Wellness     220

Twenty Seven:     A Final Story     229

# Simple Moves

# For the

# Body & Soul

Introduction

Health + Fitness = Life

That's what life's about; right? If only we could achieve it easily! As humans, we tend to do a greater number of things the hard way, than the easy way.

(We do tend to approach things in a backwards fashion)

Though we eat out frequently, we do try to eat healthy: Charbroiled Chicken Burgers; Sushi; Salad Bars; even Mc Donald's and Subway have created healthy menus. Fitness Centers have increased in popularity: Curves; 24 hour Fitness; Gold's Gym. And, Weight Loss Centers have popped on every corner: Jenny Craig; Weight Watchers.

Our bodies have no excuse for lack of fitness. Of course, our schedules are a bit hectic with: work; soccer games; piano practice; birthday parties; social events, etc. We work ten to twelve hour days, while our children are farmed out to strangers, for their care. Is there really any time for fitness? Let's see, now ~~ oh, yes, I have a 5:00AM opening; I will schedule in fitness. And, rain or shine, I'll be up before dawn to take care of me.

Sounds like a good plan, doesn't it? Well, have you heard the saying "The best laid plans of mice & men"? We have good intentions.

When was the last time your good intentions really got anything done? No, they are just that 'good intentions'. The great plan to take care of one's self got lost along the path of life. Oh, it might have worked well for the first few days; maybe even a week or two; at best, a couple of months, if getting fit fell on your list of New Year's resolutions.

By mid ~ year, life had caught up with us. The seasons changed; daily schedules began an hour earlier; and ended an hour later. Before long, sleep was much sweeter than a morning work out. "I'll just skip this one day" we told our selves; promising we would make it up tomorrow. Are you still waiting for that 'tomorrow' day to come around? I know I'm guilty of it!

We've become a lazydasical society, haven't we? Putting off for today the things we can do tomorrow sounded pretty good, earlier in life. Now, it's catching up with today. The present is the here and now. The past we can never recover. So, we make yet another New Year's resolution of fitness first. "This year, I'm going to stick to it!" Now, I don't mean to sound cynical, here, but isn't that what you said last year? Silly me; my mistake.

Let's rewrite the equation to a formula we can better relate to. In doing so, we can break down all aspects of the equation.

Instead of: Health + Fitness = Life; let's do: Health + Laughter + Fitness + Soul = Life. Now, we have an equation we can work with.

The four basic groups can be broken down to include sub groups, and we can stay on track with our discussion. Through the following chapters we will share recipes for better health; and a laugh or two; as you become reacquainted with 'Simple Moves for the Body & Soul.
*(Now, I feel better about this; how about you?)*

# Chapter

# One

## *The Connection of Body, Mind and Heart*

The mind; the brain is located within the head, at the top of the human body. It was not placed at our feet, to be trodden or cut off. The mind was given an elite position: at the top of our body. Yes, this was by masterful design: Placed right at the top, to be the leader of the pact. A quick thinker, the brain is the first one to see all things.

The brain tells the body what to do; when to do it; why it needs to be done; and how to accomplish the task at hand. It tells us when we feel hot; cold; if we're injured; doing things the right (or wrong) way. The brain makes decisions; plans our day; tells us when to smile; laugh; or cry.

There is a direct line between our heart and our brain. They work well together. The heart beats and the brain thinks; what an awesome combination. Could mankind create such a mechanism? Not on his own! We might copy the imagery, but, creating the model took a much higher power.

With this, we see the connection of body, mind and heart. We nurture each part in a unique way. We have established the connection between the heart and the soul. Doesn't it make sense that the soul should require nurturing, also? Isn't it all part of the equation?

Yes, it is! So, what makes it so difficult to complete the equation? Is it that difficult to grip? Maybe it's presented in such a simple form that we fail to understand it. You know us humans like to complicate things.

With all the love and care given to us, I do not believe Heavenly Father would leave us hangin', here. So, what's the problem? Maybe it's the combination itself: Health + Fitness = Life. We have learned that the heart, mind, body and soul all work together. Each has their distinct function. Each has a purpose the other can not provide. Yet, mankind decides to complicate their functions.

Wait! If mankind decides; doesn't that lend fault to the brain? No, it does not. The brain is not at fault. Does that lend fault to the soul? No, it does not. It means as a whole, we must take responsibility for our actions. If we neglect one area of our lives, we can not blame its demise on another. To avoid problems, we need to take care of every unit with the same amount of enthusiasm. Does that mean I have to actually DO some thing? I have to be active? There you go again ~~ complicating things.

Keep reading: we'll fill in the blanks as we go. You will see how the body; mind; soul; health; fitness and faith add up; to equal life. Don't be scared to pick up your pen now and then and write notes in the margins, or on the back pages. If you truly want to learn some thing, just write it down.

It's amazing how that really does work! They say that when you write something down, it processes through your brain five times. Five times! We should have notebooks on our shelves instead of books; filled with our own writings.

*Okay, okay: let's get on with it.*

Making a decision, and sticking to it, is called a commitment. Yes, there's a fancy little word for that action: commitment. It requires one decision; followed by persistence. A simple equation, really: Why do we make it so difficult?

Maybe we have become a bit too accepting of unkept promises. Have we lost faith in mankind? Mankind is the only species with the ability to make a promise; and withdraw it a moment later. Is this what we have become? How do we regain the faith?

Faith: believing in something you can not touch, hear or see; the uncertain belief in some intangible thing or being; an unbreakable trust. Do we have faith in mankind? This species has let us down a time or two. Do we have faith in a higher power? Ah, I hit a nerve, did I?

There's the ticket for faith, right there: that higher power. I call my higher power 'Heavenly Father': My God; my creator; my life line; my strength. How do you refer to your higher power? Where does your strength come from? Maybe you believe we create our own existence.

Whatever your belief, let's presume (for lack of argument) that we all have a higher power. The very breathe within each of us is decided upon by some one or some thing we can not touch or see. Our ears can not hear their voice.

Our life is out of our control. The sun rises and sets on command from this power. The earth rumbles; the waves explode; the wind blows: by one command. Mankind refers to it as 'mother nature'; an act of God.

If his power is so eminent in the realm of nature, wouldn't that power be a part of our make up, as well? Is it realistic to believe that the same power controlling the elements of the Earth would control the elements of my being? When I look in the mirror, I see a being created by a higher power. I see a reflection of goodness; compassion; and tender love; A truly magnificent piece of art. I believe it to be so.

This handmade work of art was (once upon a time) perfect. Then it came to Earth: the imperfect place. With its attitudes and elements, the world ate away at the soul of this being. The years and tears and solitude gave way for lack of faith. The higher power of my existence did not give up on me. He never lost hope in my return. He gave me life; breathe; love; family & friends. He gave me his word, to help me grow; learn; and gain a new perspective on life. He gave me a heart to feel love; hurt; compassion and kindness.

If the heart is the soul; the soul is the center of the body. The physical body requires food, water, nutrition, cleansing. Without these, the body becomes weak, afflicted and dirty. The body can not manage these tasks with out help from the mind. The mind speaks to the body's parts, and they fulfill the tasks on command.

Maybe command is a harsh word to use, here. The mind does not command. The body and mind are a team; companions. They work on the element of respect; not authority.

Respect is a seven letter word. Seven is a number that stands alone; yet, works well with others. With its head held high, the number seven stands up right, leaning slightly. This shifts the weight of its body so it is evenly balanced. Though tall and strong, he is not arrogant or demanding. No, he is of a kind and gentle design. Say it: seven.

The sound of his name is can not be taken as rude or obnoxious, either. Say it, again: seven. Yes, it does sound rather nice. So, you think this is silliness? Try saying eight; nine; or ten. Go ahead, no one is listening. Even if they are; they will most likely think you are doing an important exercise. Who knows, this may be contagious!

Now, did you hear the difference in the sound of each number? Ten is often held in high degree. Like: pick a number between one and ten; one being the lowest; ten the highest. Have you ever been asked to measure pain?

The number ten is always associated with the strongest amount of pain. The number eight is like the start of a new week. Since there are only seven days in a week; number eight is like a first born child. He has bragging rights. Number nine is in the 'top three'; she gets to the best of both worlds.

# Chapter Two

### *First, Let's Talk About health.*

A healthy body is a must in life. Some of us learn this truth earlier than others. Some people just never learn. Our health is affected, in part, by: the things we do; foods we eat; environments we live and work in; our family life; and social status. While some of these factors are avoidable; some are out of our control. For each of us, life is different.

### *Things We Do:*

Most of us begin this life in a fairly healthy state. Our youth is spent learning about all the ups and downs we should expect along the way. As we make it through those 'dare devil' days, we begin to think we are a bit invincible. (Yes, you know you did) We over indulged in pizza; ice cream; candy and Kool ~ Aid. When our bellies had a fit (we felt a bit sick) we turned to mom & dad for a quick relief.

In our teens, we became all too aware of our hormones and progesterone. Some learned promiscuity; a few believed in saving themselves for marriage; others claimed celibacy; or a gay or lesbian lifestyle. With the mix of diseases out there, it's incredible any one has relations prior to seeing a certificate of good health from participating parties.

We're not talking about mild stuff, here. No, we have Aids; HIV; Hepatitis; and a grip of venereal diseases. We have seen more 'relations' deaths in the past thirty years than my mother saw in her entire lifetime. It's no wonder condoms are sold in the supermarket!

We learn how to work hard and get far too little sleep. Our date books are full and, with the blink of an eye, play time is all but lost. So, we learned to play just as hard. Now, the way I see it, if a guy works hard; plays hard; and resists sleep; he's asking for a quick burn out. (Or a heart attack)

What happened to the need for balance? Did we become super human along the way? If so; I got gypped! Point me toward the guy who hands out those super powers.

Well, the body isn't made to perform at maximum speed with out proper rest. It's part of the balance of things. Health advocates recommend at least six to eight hours of sleep per day. Without proper rest, our bodies get tired. Consequently, we run our selves full speed ahead into exhaustion.

Then, we race to the doctor and demand a pill to boost our energy. When the pills fail to meet our expectations, we blame the doctor. If a pill is the answer; we are really in trouble. There are only twenty four hours in a day. What ever happened to personal responsibility?

If our own life styles did not affect our health, we could depend on those around us to fill in the gaps. In the sixties and seventies, people lived rather risqué lives. Television shows portrayed 'the good life' as days of Cigars; Martinis; and Penthouses. Who wouldn't want that kind of life? Commerce didn't mind: Cigarette sales were on the rise.

Alcohol sales increased; and glitz and glitter were of high demand. You did not have to be a smoker to be introduced to the smoke. Medical Experts have linked second hand smoke to several lung diseases; including cancer.

By mid ~ life, our eyes were blurred; joints were aching; and we had spasms in muscles we never knew existed. After nine holes on the golf course with the chiropractor, he put your back in place at no charge. Some times it pays to let him beat you at the game, know what I mean?

With the physician on speed dial, it was safe to join the adult baseball team. How did you ever hold on to that ball? With that collection of pill bottles requiring 'easy caps'; it must have been a struggle.

With my experience in Home Health Care, it was expected that I would be the one to care for my folks, as they aged. Recently, my father went to the doctor to complain about his woes. Some were actually justified; while others could have been avoided.

Fortunately, I knew the regimen. As my father chewed out his doctor for not helping him get rid of this, that, and the other, I bit my tongue. How can you help some one who doesn't follow your advice?

This nice young doctor listened, patiently, while dad gave him the what ~ for. When the coast was clear, the doctor said "Have you been taking this & that the way I told you to?" "I'm not taking any more pills" Dad retorted. Finally, I rudely interrupted. "Dad" I said "How do you expect him to help you, if you won't follow his advice?" The room was quiet, for a moment.

Dad now follows doctor's orders; and, feeling better! Aside from medical issues, life continued on. Weekends were farther apart, since the kids were grown. When they were home, we could count on them to wake us up in the morning. They never got the hang of sleeping in on Saturdays. Crazy kids: up all night (Friday Night); awake at the break of day on Saturday. They must belong to the neighbor, 'cause they didn't learn that from us! We finally replaced the alarm clock. Yeah, that day the snooze button didn't work, and you were late for a meeting with your new boss man. That was impressive.

One night you decide to take your spouse to dinner and a movie. It's been a while since the two of you had a night on the town. Maybe you'll do some dancing afterwards. As you wait for a table, you notice the new menu prices. Your spouse says 'No Way'; they are not about to pay those prices: highway robbery! Sizzler's is lookin' pretty good.

By the time you arrive out side the theatre, you have five minutes to park the car and get inside. Finally, the movie begins; and all you can say is: Thank goodness for short lines, and magnifying glasses!

Okay, so we didn't take as good a care of our bodies as we imagined. Now we understand why we were told: 'stop running in the house; look both ways; and turn down the music'. With a hearing aide in each ear, we still can't hear what's being said. Though I have noticed it's easier to hear across the room than to hear a sound close by. Being tone deaf is not any fun.

Nowadays, the floor is much farther away, leaving one's feet to feel rather neglected. Those rough spots on the heels keep coming back to visit, and the toe nails are way too long. Those bunions weren't there last week, either.

Thank goodness for the massive number of nail shops around town. Most are fairly inexpensive and accept drop in and last minute customers, so appointments don't need to be made (or broken). Lord knows we have enough of those on our calendars, already.

Remember, it's important to cancel medical appointments a day ahead, or you could be charged for the office visit. (Or more)

The last trip to the barber shop was almost an insult to the barber. With hair too thin to comb, he recommended a shave. Not my beard, silly: the top of my head! Problem is: if he shaves my head, he'll have to trim my beard. Now, I know it's getting way too long, 'cause the neighborhood kids mistook me for Santa Claus. I'm sure the adults (must have) warned us about the dangers of life; it's just not fresh in the 'ol memory bank.

With the economy in a rut, it's best to do things our self, when possible. If you can shave your own head; by all means, do it your self. Just be really careful, okay? A cut on your head could land you in the emergency room instead of on the dance floor. (Get my drift?)

Use safety and caution when self ~ diagnosing; attempting do ~ it ~ your self projects; and taking short cuts. The out come could be more costly than having a professional do the job.

# Chapter

# Three

***Things We Should Do:***

Though it was imperative he take one extra pill each day, my father was right in his quest to forego adding to his collection. Too often pills are added automatically. How many meds do you take? If you are over fifty, chances are you take one or two; maybe more. We often self~diagnose, adding over the counter remedies to our stash of 'cure alls'. On each package is written 'check with your physician before taking this'. Raise your hand if you did not check with your doctor, first. That's what I thought!

Unfortunately, this could lead to serious health issues. In some cases; death has been reported. Not all medications are interactive. Though we may be wise to many things, we need to remember our level of expertise. Your pharmacist can be a great help in selecting over the counter remedies. For best results, remember, too, to make sure you tell them ALL of the meds you are taking.

For quick access, make a list of current meds and keep it in your wallet. Include all over the counter items such as: Aspirin; inhalers; cough syrups; Tylenol. Add a special section listing any allergies you may have. This will help the pharmacist choose the best remedy for your issues. By the way, this could also save your life in an emergency.

The next time you visit your doctor, show him your list of current meds, including over the counter remedies. Make sure he is aware of any allergies you have. If you have blood pressure issues (most of us do), this will be extremely helpful information. Do not assume your health care professionals are mind readers.

Make a list of questions or concerns you wish to discuss with them, a few days ahead of time. Even if you have a great memory, it's easy to get caught up in the moment and forget to address the issues. Yes, this is experience speaking, once again.

Do you think young people will ever learn from the mistakes others? No, I guess not. The simple things in life seem to be the most difficult to perceive. Humans are hard headed and stubborn creatures.

And, to think we expect our offspring to accept things so readily. Yet, what they do not learn from home, they will learn from the world.

So, we need to keep telling them, anyway. Be the base for their earthly education. They may never admit it, but they will appreciate your efforts. Who knows, one day that might realize just how intelligent you truly are. (Miracles do happen) While you're at it; tell them about shopping for groceries & the downside to fast foods, as well.

Good health is dependent upon every aspect of our lives. Regardless of race; social status or finances, each of us is susceptible to health issues. Stress plays a large part in defining our health. It is the culprit to many health problems.

Heart Disease; High Blood Pressure; Psoriasis; Bloating; Anxiety; Colds; are all associated with stress. Stress affects our work; home life; attitude; relationships and success or failures. What can we do to prevent it?

Breathe. Just Breathe. Now, take a step back from the situation, and reevaluate things. Sounds easy enough, doesn't it? And, yes, it is often a bit more complicated than that. However, when we take a moment to reassess a situation, our mind is forced to take a second look, also. For just a moment, we bind the negative energy and release a much more valuable energy: positive energy.

Our tempers can be controlled, if we choose to control it. Unfortunately, it is much easier to release the negative energy, than it is to bind it. Some people blame their 'hot heads' on their heritage. The German's and Irish are typical hot heads. The English are prudes. The French, romantic; and Italians speak in loud tones. Well, I hate to be the one to break it to you ~~ each of us has these qualities; regardless of our heritage.

If you need an avenue to vent, some say "Get a pet". Pets are great listeners. The sound of your voice intrigues them. When you laugh, they get excited. When you cry, they are truly concerned. A pet's arms can not hold you, or help you out of a jam. Instead, they set beside you or on your lap and snuggle up to help console their friend. Please be kind to your pet: they do not anger as we do.

A pet longs for your kindness. They love you, and want to protect you; unconditionally. Your pet does require care. Your veterinarian may recommend a special diet or exercise program, as well. Pet stores carry a variety of nutritional products, toys and treats, and care products for all your pet's needs. Remember, too: pets should have a good bath and have their toe nails trimmed regularly. Most pet stores offer this service.

## *Recipes for Better Health*

1. Communicate with your physician and follow Medical Advice
2. Get plenty of rest. Some things may have to wait for tomorrow
3. Exercise within your capabilities. (we have a few tips; read on)
4. Control your tongue. You will accomplish more with a cup of sugar than you will with a drop of vinegar. Practice virtue
5. Realize you are NOT super human. Allow others to help. Let them be blessed
6. Make decisions. Decide within your heart; not with your mind
7. Keep promises. Don't make promises you do not intend to keep
8. Breathe. Just breathe. Find a quiet place and rejuvenate
9. Get a pet. (If you can) Trust me, they help reduce stress
10. Regain your faith. Higher power or energy: listen with your heart

*Chapter*

*Four*

## The Food We Eat:

When I was young, my parents were big advocates of eating balanced meals. We raised our own vegetables; picked fruit straight off the trees (yes, in the fields); and had fresh milk, eggs, and cheese delivered to our front door every other morning. Our tomatoes and herbs were grown in our own backyard; no extra chemicals or hot houses.

We didn't have a lot of money, so we couldn't run to town on a whim. My folks grew up in the depression era, so they knew how to save a buck. Though we didn't have a lot of money; we never went with out. We had seven mouths to feed; plus mom & dad. Canned vegetables meant we had picked, cleaned, and canned them our selves. Mom did buy bread. (Thank Heaven's!)

Now, I promise not to tell you how I shoveled snow; or walked two miles to school; or woke before dawn to milk the cows: that's my folks' story. We did live about ten miles outside of town. We grew up in a farming community where neighbors took care of one another. Everyone did their part. Growing a garden meant you always had fresh produce to share with the neighborhood.

Today's produce is picked green; hot house harvested; sent across the country; kept in cold storage to 'ripen'; and sold all across the country as 'fresh'. Doesn't the term 'fresh' imply the produce was removed from the fields within the past few days? Or, is that just my mistake? Silly me; I get confused on these matters, don't I?

Now, I was raised in Northern California. We lived across the street from a huge peach orchard. Through the years, I had become quite an expert on the subject. We picked, canned, flash froze and ate more peaches than most people I know, today.

Friends gave us lug boxes filled with cling and freestone peaches. Believe me; we had nightmares about peaches chasing us around the room with a pitter in their clenched fist. Not a pretty sight!

The next time you go through a produce aisle, stop and check out the fruits and veggies. You decide how 'fresh' they really are. Now, in today's market, some items are grown as organic. I noticed they often leave the vines attached to these organic tomatoes. That's impressive! You can actually smell the difference. Go ahead and try it; don't just take my word for it.

Several years ago, I took a trip to Texas, to visit my sister, Jean. On the way home from the airport, Jean said she needed to stop at the market for a few things. Not just any store would do, for my sister. She only shopped at 'the best' stores. (H.E.B.) Dad always said "If you want quality, shop at quality stores". Jean took heed to his words.

We entered the store near the produce section. Jean grabbed a cart, and waltzed right past the fresh peaches. As she reached for her produce, I said "What are these?" "Peaches" she replied. "PEACHES?" I must have said a bit louder than intended, because all eyes were on me. Poor Jean was so embarrassed.

"I can't believe you said that" she said with a stern voice (giggling under her breathe). "I can't believe they call those things peaches!" I said (a bit quieter). As I glanced around the room, I spotted four men staring at me with an unpleasant look. "That's the entire produce management" Jean must have seen them, also. She didn't let me shop with her often.

Well, what did you expect from a 'peach expert', anyway? I learned a big lesson that day: not every thing in Texas is big! The store was a quality store by every measure they could achieve. I'll say that much for it. It was clean; well stocked; and the employees were friendly and helpful. And, there peaches were not from California!

Going to the supermarket is unavoidable. Everything we consume is purchased through a supermarket. Our meat; vegetables; fruit; dairy products; pet food; cleaning supplies and pet food are found below one roof. Some stores (Target; Fred Meyer) offer groceries; house wares; electronics and clothing. With super stores on the rise (Wal ~ Mart), we can now service our vehicles while we shop for groceries.

Day after day, we are warned against buying one product or another. Either lead levels are too high or products don't hold up. Food products around the world have been removed from grocery stores due to tainted contents. Are these unsafe products shipped from around the world? Or, do the bulk of the items appear to come from one or two countries? Maybe we should pay attention to the information on the labels.

As you walk along the canned foods section, stop and look at a label or two. The Food and Drug Administration requires the canning companies to list all ingredients on their labels. Are you on a low ~ salt diet? You might want to give those labels an extra look. Most canned foods have salt added, as a preservative. Yes, you can rinse off most of it. However, you may loose some of the flavor, as well. Check it out; and give it a try. Don't just take my word for it. (I don't make this stuff up)

Are you a quick ~ chef? You know: the kind that buys microwavable foods; frozen dinners; boxed pastas. Have you read the back of the box, lately? Interesting ingredients, don't you think? Just how many of those words can you actually pronounce? I quit trying. If we knew what they were, we might just pass it by. When looking for low fat products, keep in mind most low fat foods are higher in sodium. Check it out.

Somewhere along the way, we began to realize that Mc Donald's and Pizza Hut do not offer the healthy menus we need to sustain good health. So, we switched to Carl's Jr. (char broiled burgers); Subway (healthy choice subs); and Sizzler's (great salad bar). We ate as much and as often as we liked. Eating out became all too easy. When was the last time you actually cooked for your self or family?

No, boxed, frozen or microwave meals do not count. I'm talking about good old fashioned home cooking. You know, the kind requires a few minutes to prepare: cut vegetables, cook meats, boil water or keep an eye on the oven. Yes, like our past generations did.

Have you noticed how well they lived? Even the poor had better health than the richer families of today. There was always food on the table. They grew their own vegetables and raised their own meat. No preservatives necessary for fresh foods.

As our days get busier, we rely on simplicity more and more. Much like our forefathers, we look for nutritious, healthy meals. Recipe books are plentiful, yet we put them in out of reach places. (Like the top shelf) On that rare occasion that you prepare one of the meals, you realize one or two ingredients are missing from your pantry. By the time you start the preparations, you're wishing dinner was ready to put on the table.

Don't fret: you are not alone. Most of us do our meals the same way. It's frustrating, and often finds us rushed and irritated. Here's an idea: Next time you make a meatloaf, make two. Put one in the oven; the other one goes in the freezer. Several dishes can be made ahead and kept in the freezer for about a month or two. These are not 'left over' or frozen dinners. Each meal was pre planned by you, and made fresh. No preservatives.

Once you get in the habit of doing 'make ahead' meals, you will find your self shopping more efficiently, and spending a lot less time in the kitchen. The family just might enjoy helping, too! I like to pre cook most of my meals. Then, if I forget to take it out of the freezer to thaw, I can just pop it in the microwave.

Get to know that defrost button; then reheat in the microwave or conventional oven. Let the family help by making a salad; biscuits, and setting the table. By the time everything is ready, dinner goes on the table in a short amount of time, and the stress has turned to laughter and conversation.

Initially, taking time to read labels may seem too time intensive. It does take a few extra minutes to do this. Relax; breathe; and focus on the task at hand: selecting healthier foods for your family. To help you in your quest, we have compiled an A to Z list of foods, along with ideas on how to incorporate them into your diet.

# Chapter

# Five

## *Our A to Z List of Feel ~ Good Foods*

*A = Almonds:* Are the best nut source for Vitamin E, an antioxidant; also loaded with heart ~ healthy mono ~ and polyunsaturated fats. Try Thai peanut sauce or a PBJ with almond butter instead of peanut butter.

*B = Berries:* Dubbed as 'super food' berries help lower blood pressure; increase the body's level of good cholesterol (HDL); and contain protein antioxidants. A great low ~ calorie snack; packed with fiber. Add to yogurt, cereal, and salads. Use frozen raspberries as the chilling ingredient for smoothies.

*C = Cabbage:* Cabbage and its botanical relatives contain potentially cancer ~ fighting compounds called Glucosinolates. Red cabbage gets its red ~ purple color from the powerful antioxidants Anthocyanin, Add to soups; stir fries; and sandwiches.

*D = Dates:* At a mere 66 calories, just one caramel ~ sweet Medjool date can satisfy a dessert craving. A good source of fiber, too. We found moist Medjools in California's Coachella Valley.

*E = Eggs:* Research shows eggs got a bad rap in the past. For most people, eggs may actually be good for the heart. They're also full of protein, low in calories and a good source of lutein and zeaxanthin; pigments that may keep your eyes healthy. Try this: add eggs to a sautéed mixture of tomatoes, bell peppers, onions and olive oil. When done, top with cheese.

*F = Fat:* Surprise: Some fats may actually be good for you. Fat helps the body process carbs and proteins. Cooking with mono ~ and polyunsaturated fats adds flavor and texture; its satiating effects can also keep you from over eating. Don't over do it; small amounts of fat only. Tip: no more than 30 % of your daily calories should come from fats. Choose unsaturated olive, canola, and nut oils.

*G = Grass ~ Fed:* Nature knows best. Meat from cows and sheep are lower in fat and cholesterol, and higher in beneficial omega ~ 3 fatty acids when they are allowed to graze on grass. Look for meats labeled 'grass ~ fed' or 'pasture ~ fed'.

*H = Herbs:* A great way to add fresh flavor to foods. Herbs provide bonus vitamins and minerals. Try this: In a salad, set aside some of the lettuce and add basil, cilantro, mint, or parsley lettuce in its place.

*I = Identify:* Where is your food coming from, and what is in it? In this day and age, of food ~ bourn illnesses, and questionable food ~ raising practices, it's a smart thing to do. Check the labels and identify. Ask: A good grocer will track down the answers for you.

*J = Juice:* Blend juiced vegetables in tasty combinations. A refreshing alternative to fruit juices, they're an easy way to up your daily vitamin intake. 100 % vegetable juice is also available in your grocer's refrigerator section.

*K = Kumquats:* These little citrus fruit cuties are sour on the inside, with sweet, edible skins; high in vitamin C and dietary fiber. Add sliced kumquats to your cereal, pack in your lunch, or for an on ~ the ~ go ~ snack.

*L = Lentils:* Nick ~ named the 'poster child' for healthy food, they are high in protein, fiber, 6 vitamins, folate and iron; Also low in fat ~ and cheap. This mild, Earthy variety keeps it's tiny round shape when cooked.

*M = Mustard Greens:* Loaded with vitamins A, C, and K, mustard greens have a pungent bite and cook to tenderness in just a few minutes. Try this: sauté with garlic, then scramble in a few eggs, and chili flakes; Makes a last ~ minute supper.

*N = Nori:* This well kept secret is actually paper ~ thin, dried seaweed. With its briny flavor, Nori is proud of its omega 3 content. Using it: cut into slivers and sprinkle on soups; stir into steamed brown rice. Adds flavor with out adding calories.

*O = Oranges:* Craving a cold glass of O.J.? Consider munching on sections of a whole orange, instead. You will benefit from almost the same amount of vitamin C; and nine times as much fiber. Pair a dish of yogurt with chopped oranges, toasted almonds, and coconut.

*P = Papaya:* This sweet, tropical fruit matches oranges, cup for cup, in vitamin C; and provides extra vitamin A. To serve: cut in wedges; serve with a squeeze of lime or in lemonade with a pinch of cayenne.

*Q = Quinoa:* (kee ~ nah)This grain ~ like seed is gluten free; high in protein; and full of vitamins and minerals (folate, iron, magnesium, and manganese). Substitute for rice or pasta.

*R = Raw:* To add texture and flavor to your side dishes, add a few raw vegetables to their cooked companions. Mix ~ up: cook pasta or rice; toss with a few raw vegetables; and top with your favorite vinaigrette dressing.

*S = Salad:* Not just a side dish; salads are great as a meal. Enjoy a Caesar; Cobb; Crab Louie; or Chef's Salad. Tip: The darker your salad greens; the more vitamins they have. (Romaine, Spinach, Watercress)

*T = Tea:* Fresh brewed is best. Its polyphenols (antioxidants) may help to lower the risk of cancer. Plus, it may help to reduce the risk of developing Parkinson's disease. Tip: A bit of lemon adds extra antioxidants.

*U = Use a smaller plate* …. Need we say more? (Yes, this really does help)

*V = Vegetarian:* Eating lots of fruits and vegetables not only reduces your risk for cancer, heart disease, and diabetes; it helps reduce the waistline, too. Carnivores need not worry: just skip one per week (from meat).

*W = Water:* Essential for life, water helps to lubricate joints, lets the body maintain the proper temperature, and flushes waste. To jazz it up, add a slice of lemon, lime, or cucumber; serve iced.

*X = X this off your list ~ fad diets.* Good diets are based on eating in moderation. Fad diets are not nutritionally sound ~ ever. Instead: focus on limiting portions; consuming more vegetables (fresh is best); and exercise.

Y = Yogurt: True or False: All yogurts are equally nutritious. (False) Some contain sugar. Studies suggest yogurt in a diet helps to regulate digestion; also a great source of calcium and protein. Look for unsweetened; with out thickeners. Mix in a fruit; a natural sweetener.

Z = *Zinfandel:* A favorite of many wine connoisseurs, it's full ~ bodied; aromatic; and, in moderation, is actually good for you. Two antioxidants in wine: resveratrol and catechins. Surprise: Wine has links to heart health. Great with apples and sharp cheese; sweet & spicy toasted nuts.

# Chapter

# Six

### *Healthy Recipes & Creative Cooking*

Now that you know the A to Z's of healthy eating, put it to work. We've put together a collection of recipes for the entire family's enjoyment. We don't like to spend hours in the kitchen ~~ so, we won't ask you to.

If you have fresh ingredients on hand, use them up, first. Meats should be thawed; vegetables should be ready to use (frozen is okay, in most cases). Be sure to read the recipe completely. Cut, divide and measure all ingredients prior to mixing. This will save time and anxiety, as you go.

If you are a creative cook, we'd love to hear your ideas for 'mixing up' these recipes. With so little family time, taking the opportunity to fix a healthy meal together makes a big difference in everyone's day; And, in their lives.

## Spinach and Persimmon Salad

*Great side to rich foods!*  
¼ cup rice vinegar  
2 Tbsp orange marmalade  
1 tsp toasted sesame oil  
Salt and ground black pepper  

5 qts baby spinach (1 ¼ lbs)  
Rinse; chill until crisp  
5 firm persimmons (5 oz ea)  
Peel; slice into wedges  
1 ½ cups glazed pecans*

In a large bowl, mix vinegar, marmalade, and sesame oil. Add salt and pepper to taste. Mix in spinach, persimmons, and pecans.

*\*Find glazed pecans in the nut section of your supermarket*

An All ~ Time Favorite Meal includes: Meatloaf; Baked Potatoes; Broccoli; Refrigerator Rolls and a Green Salad. Here's how we put it all together in about an hour.

### *Meatloaf*

*Ingredients & Directions*

| | |
|---|---|
| 3 lbs ground beef, uncooked | Add to taste: |
| 1 large onion, chopped | Garlic powder or salt |
| 3 large eggs, slightly beaten | Italian Seasoning |
| 1 cup oatmeal, raw | Salt & Pepper |
|    (Quick or Regular) | Catsup (if desired) |
| 1 cup milk | |

Preheat oven to 350° F.

In a large bowl, break up ground beef. Add onion, eggs, oatmeal, milk, and desired seasonings. Mix well, using your hands. Press mixture into a 9 x 11 baking dish. Cover with catsup, if desired. Cover dish with foil and place in oven, so allowing room for potatoes. Bake for 50 – 60 minutes.

Wash potatoes, and pierce with a fork or knife (three times per side). Wrap each potato with foil and place along side baking dish. Check potatoes same as meatloaf (below).

Meanwhile, in a medium to large bowl, prepare salad using your favorite ingredients. Cover with a damp paper towel, and set in refrigerator to chill. If you will be serving a vegetable, begin getting it ready, now.

Most fresh vegetables are added to a 3 quart pan of boiling water (about ½ to ¾ full). The water should just cover the top of your vegetables. Bring water back to boil, cover and cook until almost tender, about 10 minutes.

To check if meatloaf is done, insert a flat blade knife into the center of the meat. If it comes out clean, the meatloaf is done. If not, cook for another 10 minutes, and recheck. When done, remove from oven.

Increase oven heat to 400° F. Arrange biscuits in round baking pan and cook as directed. (Usually, 8 to 10 minutes) While biscuits are baking: Set table. Remove salad from refrigerator. Remove paper towel. Place a towel in a basket or medium size bowl. Place drained vegetables in a bowl.

Cut meatloaf and place sections on a serving platter. Set on table, along side your favorite dressings and extra catsup, if desired. When biscuits are done, toss them into the basket (bowl) and set on the table. Enjoy!

*Uh oh: Unexpected company will be joining you for supper. No, don't stress: Add a Quick & Easy soup!*

### Quick & Easy Vegetable Noodle Soup

| | |
|---|---|
| 1 can green beans | 1 Tbsp each: garlic powder; onion powder; parsley; Italian seasonings |
| 1 can corn | |
| 2 ½ cups egg noodles | |
| Salt; Pepper & | ½ Tbsp Tarragon |
| Bouillon to taste | Water: to cover pasta |

Bring water to boil in a large pot. Add noodles and seasonings, salt, pepper and your favorite bouillon; return to boil; reduce heat; cook pasta as directed; add vegetables; simmer a few minutes to heat veggies. Add 1 ½ cups chicken, beef or pork (cubed, shredded, or diced), if desired.

Occasionally, even the healthiest of eaters have cravings for salty; sugary; or greasy foods. Though we try to keep a balance, sometimes we cut out a little too much of one thing or another. Managing our health isn't as easy as it appears to be. It can be quite a challenge to figure out just what our body needs; each step of the way.

Maybe the weather or changes in our activities have required a greater amount of one source than we have given. For instance: in warm months our bodies need a little more salt (helps reduce legs cramps).

Our body burns calories, sugars, carbohydrates and proteins in different ways. The balance of these components depends on our level of activity. For participating in high energy sports (football; tennis; track) our body needs a larger dose of carbohydrates such as: Pancakes before football practice; burgers for the basketball court; or bagels & cream cheese before a tennis match. Try it: You might just improve your game.

One of our favorite meals is a single ~ pot chicken dish. The list of ingredients is not amount specific. The variation depends on your family's size; taste buds; and the size of frying pan used. We used a Wok for the number of items listed.

### *Sautéed Chicken with Vegetables & Herbs*

*Ingredients & Directions:*

| | |
|---|---|
| 3 to 4 chicken breasts | 4 stalks celery, chunked |
| 16 baby red potatoes | 16 baby carrots |
| 1 medium onion, sliced | 2 Tbsp parsley |
| 2 Tbsp garlic powder | 3 Tbsp Olive oil |
| 2 Tbsp ground pepper | 4 Tbsp flour |
| 4 Tbsp Corn Starch | Water |

Divide seasonings in half. Combine flour to one half of seasonings, and coat the chicken with the flour mixture. In a Wok, heat oil (med high); brown chicken, lightly, on each side, remove from pan. Add onion, celery, carrots, potatoes to the Wok, and about 4 cups water. Top with chicken. Sprinkle with remaining seasoning. Add enough water to cover vegetables. Cover; cook 15 to 20 minutes at slow boil, stirring occasionally. Reduce heat to medium, if needed. Add water, as needed to maintain fluid level. When chicken is done, remove chicken and vegetables; set aside. Put corn starch in a coffee mug and add 1 cup hot broth, stirring quickly. Slowly return the mixture to the Wok, stirring constantly. Great over pasta; Serve with hot rolls.

# Chapter Seven

## *A few Quick & Easy Ideas*

### **Chili Salad**

| *Ingredients & Directions:* | *Optional Ingredients:* |
| --- | --- |
| 2 cans chili, heated | *Sour cream* |
| 1 large package Fritos | *Chives* |
| 1 package (8 oz) cheese | *Guacamole* |
| 2 large tomatoes, chopped | *Jalapenos* |
| 1/3 head lettuce, shredded | Hot sauce or taco sauce |

Put Fritos in individual soup bowls. Cover with chili. Sprinkle with cheese, tomatoes and lettuce. If desired, add optional ingredients. Serve with taco sauce.

### Crab ~ Tomato Cocktail

*Ingredients & directions:*

1 (48 oz) can tomato juice

1 small bottle catsup       ½ tsp Worcestershire Sauce

2 tsp sugar       ¼ tsp onion salt

Salt to taste       2 cans grapefruit sections

1/2 cup lemon juice       2 large cans crabmeat

Prepare 8 hrs ahead. Drain grapefruit; Mix all ingredients; Spoon into punch cups. Serve with wheat thins and slice of lemon, if desired.

### Stove ~ Top Spanish Rice Casserole

*Ingredients & Directions:*

1 lb ground beef       1 cup * rice, uncooked

1 medium onion, chopped       2 cups * water

1 bell pepper, chopped       *If using instant rice, use*

1 large can stewed tomatoes       *2 cups rice and 2 cups*

1 pkg Taco Seasoning       *water*

Brown ground beef, onion and bell pepper; drain off fat. Mix remaining ingredients, including rice; adding salt and pepper to taste. Bring to a sot boil; let simmer (covered) about 20 minutes.

## Lunch Delite

*Ingredients & Directions:*

1 can meat, diced
  (Spam; Chicken; Beef)
½ tsp minced onion
½ tsp prepared mustard
2 Tbsp Sweet Pickle Relish
3 Tbsp mayonnaise
2 hard boiled eggs
1 cup grated cheese
Hamburger buns

Mix meat, eggs (if desired), onions, mustard, relish and mayonnaise in medium bowl. Spread on hamburger buns. Top with cheese.

## Cornflake No ~ Bake Cookies

*Ingredients & Directions:*

1 cup sugar
1 cup light Karo syrup
1 ½ cup peanut butter
  (Chunky or Creamy)

6 cups corn flakes

Combine sugar and Karo syrup; bring to boil. Add peanut butter to sugar and syrup mixture. Do not cook any longer. Mix ingredients to smooth, and pour over corn flakes and mix. Spoon out onto waxed paper and let cool.

## Jet Pups *(Mini Corn Dogs)*

*Ingredients & Directions:*

| | |
|---|---|
| Pancake mix | Water |
| Corn meal | Hot dogs |
| Canned milk | Toothpicks |

Mix 4 parts pancake mix; 1 part corn meal; Dilute 2 parts canned milk to 1 parts water. Combine dry ingredients with milk and water mixture. (Batter should be heavier than regular pancake mix). Cut hot dogs into 4 pieces. Insert one toothpick into each 'mini' hot dog; Dip hot dogs into batter. Drop into 400 F oil; deep fry until golden brown; turning if needed. Cool slightly before eating. *Serve with mustard and ketchup.*

## Tacos on a Plate

*Ingredients & Directions:*

| | |
|---|---|
| 1 lb ground beef | Tomatoes, chopped |
| 1 pkg Sloppy Joe Seasoning | Lettuce, chopped |
| ( or Taco seasoning) | Cheddar cheese, grated |
| 1 (6 oz) can tomato sauce | Fritos Corn Chips, regular |
| ¼ ~ ½ cup water | Taco sauce, optional |

Brown ground beef in hot skillet. Sprinkle with seasoning mix over meat and stir in tomato sauce and water; simmer, stirring occasionally, 5 to 10 minutes. On each plate, put a handful of Fritos; spoon meat over chips. Add a layer of grated cheese, lettuce and tomato. Sprinkle with Taco sauce, if desired.* *Easier for kids to handle than tacos in a shell*

# Chapter

# Eight

***Environments we live and work in:***

As we journey through this life, we are exposed to a variety of elements. Our subways; train stations and roadways provide gases; fumes; and poor quality air flow. Even out on the highway, our air is limited to computerized air systems that can not possibly purify our air to a healthy standard.

Hard as they may try: artificial is just that: artificial. We rely on the government to issue standards. How are they doing, so far?

Work places are filled with stress: High demands for performance, perfection, and deadlines. Then, it seems we are never satisfied with our duties; title; co workers; or boss. Once upon a time, people actually stayed at the same job for 5, 10, 20 years. Today, we have this need to move forward; fast. Our patience is worn thin far too easily.

We are a tireless people, expecting more from others than we are willing to give of our selves. Passing the buck; believing our own ideas to be of much greater value than the guy beside us. We measure our selves by financial worth. Social status is everything to this growing nation. If our neighbor has less, we condemn him, or avoid him. Has it occurred to us that we may be the source of our own stress? Are we 'stewing' on matters we need to let go of?

No, I am not blaming you for all of your stress. I am blaming, in part, the life styles we have allowed to consume us. What ever happened to 'doing the best we can'? When did we start believing 'stuff' was so important to our lively hood? Gosh, keeping up with the 'Jones' is hard work! I know several people who can't seem to live their life any other way. They are so in tuned with what their neighbor has ~~ and, they will not have any thing less.

My friend, let's call him 'Mike', worked in construction for many years. In the early 1980's, Mike was summoned to build a new home for his boss, 'Jeff'. Now, Jeff and his wife had only one young daughter. Jeff's wife shared a real estate office with her mother. When Mom built a fancy new home; Jeff's wife thought they had to, also.

On a nice corner lot, Mike built this couple a 2 ~ story; 6 bedroom; 5 bath home; with sunken living room; game room; two dish washer; commercial refrigerators; and maid's quarters.

Oh, and 3 double car garages: one for him; one for her; and one for their boat. This lovely, three quarter of a million dollar home (yep, $750 K) was quite a masterpiece. (It was 1980) But, mercy me: who was going to live in it? There's just the three of them.

This was quite the showplace, back then. Remember, it was only the early 1980's. Folks would drive by and peek in the windows and gawk about. It was the new 'topic' around town, for sure. Now, when people put multiple refrigerators in their homes, don't you assume they will actually use them? You should never assume!

Jeff and his lovely wife did enjoy entertaining. In fact, they threw a pretty good sized party at least once a month. With the completion of their Olympic size swimming pool parties were held every two weeks. Yes, these appliances should have been put to good use.

Instead, every party was catered. That's right: full catering was part of the deal. You didn't think a lady of that stature would cook, did you? Honestly, I don't believe she ever knew how to cook. Her mother would not have taught her: she had two dishes washers and caterers.

Stress? No stress here; this couple had life all figured out. They didn't do the everyday things most of us do. They had a bank role; and they used it. Jeff was a hard working guy; his wife came from big money, and had a great career, and they lived life by their own rules. To some, they lived a dream life. Were they happy?

Truly, I do not believe so. About 10 years later; they divorced. They sold the big home; fought over money; and Jeff had to take a few months off work (heart trouble). Did they enjoy those ten years? Did stress play a part in their break up? Only they know the truth of it all.

The answers are none of my business. One thing's certain: they lost touch with one another along the way to success. It's a sad scenario.

# Chapter

# Nine

### *Emotional Roller Coasters*

Our emotions play a heavy part in relationships. Not just 'couple' relationships; any relationship. From the home to school; and work to friendships; emotions have a field day keeping up with us. We laugh at sad movies; cry at happy ones. A room full of people, and we feel alone; yet, a small group can be suffocating.

How confusing it all can be. With the constant need for change, our mind does not give our emotions sufficient time to adjust from one scenario to another. Our hop scotch across life leaves many unanswered questions our heart has no time to dwell on.

Ah, the heart, again. So, that's where it's been all this time ~~ playing hop scotch! For some, it's more like a roller coaster ride. They stop and start at the push of a button. As they go 'round the track, their 'seat' (temper) rises and falls on a whim. Now and then, they even jump the track. This leaves every one around them kind of 'hanging';

To wonder what will happen next. This roller coaster ride is never ending, unless they are willing to seek help (and possibly take meds). This is really hard on the 'ol ticker, man.

Yes, the heart is home to our emotions. Have you ever noticed a little 'twang' I your chest when emotions run high? You know, that invisible 'knife' that goes right through it. There's no way around it; you can't fight it; or run from it. It's there and gone in the wink of an eye. Do you see a connection, here? The heart; mind; emotions: all working in one body ~~ yours.

Maybe it's time to slow down that roller coaster you're on. If we ~~ do what? Yes! Just breathe. Unfortunately, when the roller coaster is going, so is our tongue. It lashes out at anyone and anything along the path. Breathing isn't all that tough: If only we could hold our tongue. Being one of our smallest muscles; yet, so difficult to control.

Is the need to vent so strong that we are not willing to learn how to control our tongue? If we could learn; we may be able to control our emotions. No, it does not require a push of a button.

Through out the day, we push many buttons. Our cell phones; microwaves; doorbells; and coffee makers all operate by pushing buttons. We go to work; and push buttons on the phone, computer, and elevators. The masterful minds of many unique individuals hold us captive. If we do not push the buttons; we do not progress. If we do not progress; we stand still. When was the last time you were paid to stand still?

With all of those buttons at our reach, we are able to achieve more in one day than we ever dreamed possible. Now, electronic devices are programmed by humans to provide a specific service upon command. Once we know the exact service each button represents, we simply make our selection; and wait for the device to respond. Next, we decide if we approve of the response.

If we approve, we move to the next button and continue making selections and waiting for responses until our desired out come has been satisfied. So, what happens if we push a wrong button? Wrong buttons are any button that gives a response that does not work into the equation for our desired out come.

If a conversation with someone on a roller coaster worked like our electronic devices, we could control the outcome all situations. Would life be better? Maybe yes; maybe no. I do know that it would be different.

What if we could figure out which human buttons to avoid? Maybe we could help our friends and loved ones stay off the roller coaster. Maybe we could stay on the four square pad instead of lunging down the hop scotch trail. We all have 'buttons' that get pushed in our life.

We do not have control over who or what attempts to push those buttons. We can, however, control our responses. We can give the

'Empty' signal. You know: the signal that says 'I'm sold out of temper for this or that, today. Please don't try again tomorrow; it will not be available. I'm discontinuing temper for that product'.

The grocery stores, gas stations and airports have vending machines. If a product is 'sold out' they don't forward you to another selection. No, you have to actually choose another product. This selection process takes time. You wanted a Coke. Now, you have to choose between Sprite and Dr. Pepper. If we are not interested in either of our choices, we retrieve our quarters and move on.

Imagine what might happen if we approached another individual in this same manner. Let's say I ask my husband to take me out to dinner (made a selection). He's had a hard day, and just wants to stay home (out of order). Now, I can either push another button (nag a bit); or, I can retrieve my change (accept his response) and move on (fix dinner at home). Oh, sure, I've tried it both ways. The latter has a greater long term effect.

The choices we make at each 'vending machine' in our life have an affect on our next selection. Regardless of where they are located, those vending machines are definitely related! Each has a new element of surprise (selection). Do we go here, or there; do this, that, or the other thing. Do I stay on this fast track or just slow down a bit? Will one wrong turn, or one wrong selection have that big of an affect on the rest of my life?

Maybe; Maybe not. Some are better for us than others. Elements that surround us affect our physical; emotional and spiritual well being. We play hard, work hard and get far too little sleep: Hurry; Hurry; Hurry. There's never enough hours in the day (we only have 24), and we can not borrow from tomorrow or make up for yesterday. We can only hope that our today is sufficient in the long run. Sometimes we have to adapt.

# Chapter Ten

## *Aware of the Body's Abilities*

Those born with health issues live their entire life adapting. Not because they know any other way; their way of life is all they have ever known. A person with such disabilities does not know options. There was one way to do things, and that was that.

Time is of the essence, in their world. They value each and every day. Those 24 hours they had the day before went by quickly. Today is a new day; full of promise. It can only get better!

Infants build their mind, body and strength based on their abilities. When those abilities are within normal range, choices are available for movement, fitness and growth. We walk, run, stand and move about rather freely; Limited only by our own fears. We are presented with opportunities to challenge balance, strength and knowledge. The world is ours to explore! Unless we become ill, injured or otherwise incapacitated.

When those choices are never given; they can not be taken away. If I have never fallen from a limb; I do not know how it feels to land on the ground after the fall. If I am not able to stand without support; I do not know the freedom of walking on my tip toes.

If you know the feeling of such activities, you would miss them if you were incapacitated. You can't miss what you have never known. Each day is a new adventure!

When you woke up this morning, how did you greet your new day? The first thoughts of the day help set the stage for your entire day; did you know this? So, tell me, now: Did you greet today with a smile? Or, did you say 'I'm not ready to get up yet', and crawl under your covers for a little while longer? Did you stretch like a cat, and wonder what good things might happen in your life, today? (It's okay, I won't tell!)

To be healthy, implies we are doing all we can to protect are good health. Even when we are not as healthy as we think we ought to be, we can work to preserve what we have. Limited abilities or not, we each have a responsibility to our selves to preserve the fine balance within our bodies.

Yes, our mind is acutely aware of the body's abilities. It has an understanding of our precise level of strength, growth potential, pain, and tolerance. The balance of physical and mental health must be connected. We can help!

We are going to discuss a few simple things we can do at home (safely) to help our bodies. I do not promise miracles or full youthful status. To believe we can undo all of life's wear and tear on our body is a fairytale. It took a long time to get our bodies into the shape we see today. To make a drastic change over night would cause a shock to the system. Do you think a shock to the system is healthy?

Making a change requires a decision. Not just a temporary thought change. I'm talking about a real decision: one from which we do not waver. The true, heart felt decision that we live our lives by. It's not as easy as we think it should be; Regardless of our health.

Through the years, I have cared for individuals who were: in wheelchairs; hospital beds; assisted with walkers; and fairly mobile. Is that enough to make me an expert? No! Anyone can learn to care for another. That just makes me a professional. Yes, I have learned a skill; that does not mean I know what it's like to be in your shoes.

Now, what if I told you I have been in your shoes? Okay, maybe not yours, exactly. Let me explain: Though your situation is unique from mine, I have my own history of physical disabilities from which I have learned. I have been in a wheel chair; used a walker and had to hire some one to help me 'freshen up'. After my second back surgery, I spent three months in a 'turtle brace'. It's a full brace that fits from just above the breasts to the pelvic bone.

Back braces are no fun. To get in and out of bed, the brace had to be on. I slept on an old fashioned 'fainting couch' in the living room; had a special diet, due to immobility and water retention. I could not twist or turn; walk more than fifty feet (round trip), or drive. I could not even stand long enough to do the dishes. My house was a mess; and my laundry didn't get folded the way I like it. It was not a pretty sight.

Patience is a virtue ~ good thing I have a good supply. A few years later, I was diagnosed with Rectal Cancer. Again, my house was a mess; laundry didn't get done to my liking ……. Well, you get the picture, don't you? After five weeks of chemo & radiation and five surgeries; I had the joy of five months of additional chemo.

Though the treatments did their work, I was left with 'chemo brain'. Friends & family said it looked as though I had suffered a stroke. My speech was slurred; thought patterns were off base; and I had memory issues. I was not forewarned.

The doctor said the chemo drugs would wear off after a few months. That was over five years ago. I'm still waiting for 'a few months' to pass. My balance is all out of whack: Vertigo. The medical term is Benign Positional Vertigo. The doctor said it, too, would go away in a few months time. What do you think?

If you guessed 'No'; you're right! I still have hope. It's only been about two years. It's not as much fun to get around, when your balance is off. So, you see, I have a personal understanding of the abilities and disabilities of others: Maybe not of ALL others; just a bunch.

The goal, here, is to make sure you know that we are aware of the challenges you may face in your quest for better health. How are we doing, so far? There are several issues involved with good health. If we neglect one part; we may be able to get along alright for a while. Maybe we get by for several years. The neglected part gets lost or even forgotten. Do we miss the part we are not nurturing?

Remember; the body knows its abilities. By neglecting one part of the equation, the body has been gypped. We have kept the 'easy steps' in the light. Unless we have issues that do not allow us to nurture one aspect or another, we have left those not ~ so ~ easy steps in the dark; out of sight, out of mind. We become oblivious to the dangers lurking in the dark. Maybe we should slow down. Ah, that 'slow down' thing, again.

# Chapter

# Eleven

## *Family & Social Life*

Our family and social life reflect who we are and what we believe in. From birth to adulthood, we build our character through actions and reactions to situations presented to us. Our mind is a special file cabinet which holds onto every single detail we send it.

For every decision we make, a document is created. Each document finds its way into our sub conscience (our filing cabinet). When our tempers go on a roller coaster ride, or play hop scotch we retrieve the appropriate documents to suit our emotional upheaval.

Most documents are copied to our heart, as well. No, we don't have to push extra buttons to achieve this task. This is an automatic process. It's part of the work ethics of our inner self. Not all matters are copied. The heart holds onto the most severe documents of a select group of actions: joy and heartache.

Though all documents fall into one of these categories, the heart makes a note, and appoints the filing cabinet as keeper of the less obvious matters. Be it right or wrong, every action is stamped on our heart.

How do these matters affect our sense of good health? By adding negative documents to our filing cabinet, we are prone to lose sight of the positive documents. We can not focus on negative and positive energy at the same time. A choice must be made. Yes, another one of those decisions. By choosing to dwell on the negative, we put our health at risk.

When emotions go on a ride; the mind plays tricks; and parts are left unattended. What can we do to prevent such chaos? Focusing on positive energy is the key. But, how can we achieve this goal? As the body and mind work together, they set an example for mankind. Let's take a closer look at how they work together.

## *RESPECT*

Words are our main source for communication. By giving each letter a name, we add life to the whole word. This life allows us to compare its value to our being. We will look at the encyclopedia's definition of each word's 'new name' to help in our comparisons. Just how do we measure up? Let's take a look!

## *Naming the letters:*

R = Repetitive

E = Example

S = Simultaneous

P = Polite

E = Entertaining

C = Compassionate

T = Take Turns

*Definitions:*

Repetitive: act of doing or saying some thing over and over again

Example: a person or thing to be imitated; model; precedent

Simultaneous: occurring; done; or existing together or at same time

Polite: having or showing good manner; courteous; respectful

Entertaining: interesting and pleasurable; diverting; amusing

Compassionate: sorrow for the suffering of others;
    Accompanied by an urge to help

Take Turns: to speak, do, etc. one after another in regular order

Okay, we have our definitions in order. Now, as you read the official meaning of each word, did you feel a stirring from within?

Simple little words can bring out the best in us. Did you 'puff up' a bit, believing these words were defining who you are? It's okay; I won't tell!

If you did not experience such feelings ~~ take a moment to ask your self 'Why not?' What negative elements keep your positive energy in the dark? What pain, heart break or revenge consumes you, so that peace is not allowed within?

Go ahead ~~ laugh, cry, go on a roller coaster ride ~~ what ever you need to do to free your soul. Then start again; right here. Come back to this place that freed you from your self and get on with life.

Don't 'dilly ~ dally' around; we only have one life to live. Once our time is up; we can not make it up. Just like yesterday; it's gone for good. So take just a moment, loose those chains that bind you; then move on. Make the decision to let go of all that negativity. It may be a lot easier than you think it is. No, life won't wait; now c'mon, man, we got things to do here. Time is of the essence.

If you did experience soul stirring feelings ~~ that's a good thing. Life isn't so bad, after all. Now, you may have a few dilemmas to contend with; that's alright. Part of being human is dealing with situations. We all have 'em. Those vibes you got from the definitions proved you are a good person. So, what's that got to do with any thing? I'm so glad you asked! Let's talk about that, for a moment.

Each of us has a built in desire to have others show respect for our existence. At home, we ask others to respect our privacy. In the work place, we require respect of our views; work space; privacy. We learn to respect our elders; take turns speaking (don't interrupt). Through repetition, we were being groomed for adult life.

Respect is something we earn. It is not automatic; though some believe it should be. Respect is a quiet contender. It allows us the opportunity to make something of our selves before joining our team. Certain criteria must be met before it shows it's self.

# Chapter

# Twelve

## Respect; in Layman's Terms

If we are rude or obnoxious; respect stays on the shelf. Once we settle down, and behave in a kind, and courteous manner respect jumps back into the game. We can not insist upon its presence.

Let's break this down to layman's terms. No use being complicated; life's too short to spend our energy in negative ways.

.

<u>R. E. S. P. E. C. T.</u>

*Repetitive: act of doing or saying some thing over and over again*

When you wake up in the morning, what's the very first thing you do? And you do this every day, correct? What is the last thing you do before you go to sleep, at night? This too is every day, right? Okay, now how many times a day do you pick up the phone? Do you see the connection? We are creatures of habit. We do the same things every day. Routine; repetition; schedules: call it what you like. It's all the same.

*Example: a person or thing to be imitated; model; precedent*

Whether we know it or not; like it or don't; each of us sets an example for others. Yes, Sir; each and every day. No one raises their hand to say 'Would you please set a good (or bad) example for me today, Sir?' They just stand by and watch. Our every move is being observed by some one else; young and old alike. And, you never know who is following your example; maybe a child; or your neighbor; your co workers; maybe even your boss.

*Simultaneous: occurring, done; existing together; or at same time*

Millions of people exist on our fine planet. We live; work; and play together. We co ~ exist. We do things at the same time; in the same way. For millions of people, it's: wake up at 6, out the door at 7. Our hands move the steering wheel; elevator doors open & close; the wheels on the bus go round and round ~~ all simultaneously; Like clock work.

*Polite: having or showing good manner; courteous; respectful*

When the phone rings, we say 'Hello'; a stranger sneezes, we say 'Bless You'. We open the door for another; pass in the hallway, saying 'Excuse me'; and let our elders have the last word. Elbows on the table are a 'no ~ no'; and we always chew with our mouth closed. Of course, we were raised to do this, right? Good manners were taught (and learned) by repetition.

*Entertaining: interesting and pleasurable; diverting; amusing*

On stage or off, we like to have fun. On a crowded bus, we ease the tension; first days at school are softened with a good joke; we even know how and when to engage in a (truly) meaningful conversation. Life has taught us many good lessons we enjoy sharing with others. And, we always enjoy a good laugh.

*Compassionate: sorrow for the suffering of others accompanied by an urge to help*

When sorrow fills the air, we find the blessings. Our lives are touched by those we serve. Their need is our priority. Though we can not change the world, we can offer hope and help to our neighbor. By offering a shoulder to cry on; food; shelter; a smile; we open our hearts and ease the burden of another; putting their need ahead of our own: compassion.

*Take Turns: to speak, do, etc. one after another in regular order*

Friendships; family; work; play; we live, and learn to take our turn in life. Though some are more aggressive than others, we each get our turn. We share an elevator; stairway; or cab. We speak; then listen to another. At the grocery store, we yield patience, mindful of our place in line. When others are ahead of us, we must wait our turn. Cutting the line is not an option. As patience grows, conversations are created and respect earned.

Ah, that's how it works. We have finally found the connection between us and the word. That place of mind over matter. As humans, we often think things don't really matter. Or, that too many people put their faith in the hands of others. Through this exercise, we see that things really do matter, after all. By breaking down a word, we find its purpose. It is given a life; and the definitions become clearer.

When we live life abiding by these definitions, our soul delights and health is regained. Okay, maybe it's not regained to its fullest. That was never promised. What we have is a new opportunity to move forward. We open our mind to the benefits of life: respect; health; compassion; clarity. All those elements necessary to achieve good health and fitness become clear to us.

Why are these elements so important? So glad you asked! Have you been around some one with a bad cold, lately? How was their mood? I'd bet they were not as 'chipper' as usual; And, probably not as productive, either. At work, they had difficulty concentrating; at home, they just wanted to be left alone. Is this a fair assessment?

Our emotional state has a serious impact on our physical state. It's how the body and soul work together. To obtain a positive physical being, we must exert ourselves to a positive mental being. Happy thoughts inspire a healthier body than sadness. You know, the negative brings negative syndrome. Physical vs. Emotional

The goal is to improve our Physical, Mental, and Spiritual state. The focus on our mind provides a pathway for positive decisions. The example we set forth allows others to perceive us in a positive way. This positive attitude lays a foundation for respect. Through this journey, we have grown; nurtured our minds; released the negative energy; and moved forward into a position deserving of respect from others. We earned respect.

Now, before we move on to fitness, take a moment to 'digest' what you have read. Since this may take a few minutes, set the book down (save your page); and grab a hot cup of our Magic Cocoa. The warmth of the liquid tells your brain to take a break; to relax. Set the mind at ease, first. Then, move on to the rest of your body with the fitness section. It's okay; you're only having only one cup!

### Magic Cocoa

1 cup whole milk

½ cup semisweet chocolate chips

Peppermint Stick Candy

Heat the milk over medium ~ low; don't let it boil.

Pour Chocolate Chips into an 8 ounce mug

Fill with the Hot Milk

Stir with the Candy Stick

\* Careful: this may cause a smile to appear! \*

\*\* *And, yes, kids of all ages do enjoy this!* \*\*

# Chapter

# Thirteen

***Now, Let's Talk About Fitness.***

This is a two part subject. First, you have Physical Fitness. Physical Fitness refers primarily to the physical body. It's the muscle tone; strength; and energy that give us the ability to move about (agility). The body's shell and bone structure house our organs; working hard to protect them from harm's way.

The organ's, in return, provide the necessary elements to allow the brain and body to move efficiently; like blood flow & air. The stomach alerts the brain, when it is low on food to breakdown. The brain alerts the mind and body to provide for the stomachs needs.

As we consume food and beverage products, the organs work to distribute nutrients to the appropriate areas, allowing the body to rid itself of excess. What a fine working relationship our bodies have.

The body has an unwritten list of items it needs to stay in balance. When we neglect our body's needs, it is unable to function properly.

The formula is off balance. And, you thought it was just the scales. (Silly you) A body will adapt to the formulas we provide. However, as the list of items is depleted, we are responsible for replenishing them. When we choose to make our own list, it is general in contrast to the body's needs.

Imagine this: You have returned home from the grocery store with exact ingredients for a perfect holiday meal. The turkey, dressing, seasonings, pie filling and shells are ready to go. Your kitchen cupboards are filled with items you use everyday. As the holiday arrives, you notice a few items missing: Sage; canned milk; pepper.

There's no time to go the store, so you 'make do' with what you have. Though every one raves about the meal and asks for seconds, you know it wasn't quite right. You were aware of the missing ingredients.

That's how our bodies are: aware of the missing ingredients. The body digests the food, placing nutrients where they are needed, and continuing its natural cycle. This may work seemingly well for many years. Then, one night we have difficulty sleeping. The next day we notice a lack of energy. Maybe we pull out of it; maybe we don't.

Those missing ingredients are finally catching up to us. We cooked; cleaned; and forgot to replenish our stock. The cupboards are bare. With closed cupboards, our exhausted supply went unnoticed. We were so busy accepting 'what ever would do' we did not pay attention.

One by one, those items were depleted from our stock. Bodies vs. Cupboards; Those little changes no one noticed have caught up with our body. We are feeling the effect. Fortunately, your guests will not be affected by the difference in the recipes.

Most of us have a good sense of nutrition. With our busy lives, we often get side tracked with 'cheap' options. Sometimes, we could use a little help choosing healthy foods. After weeks of searching through recipe boxes, we came up with a few yummy (easy) foods to make at home. Spend some time with the family (after supper) making these goodies. Let everyone make their favorites: they'll eat 'em up!

# Chapter

# Fourteen

## Great, Easy Recipes for A Quick Start or Snack!

### Apple Leather

| | |
|---|---|
| 3 cups applesauce | ¼ cup nuts; coarsely chop |
| ¼ tsp nutmeg | ½ cup powdered sugar |
| 1/8 tsp cinnamon | |

Combine first 4 ingredients and spread to a thickness of ½ inch in shallow pan. Bake in a moderately slow oven (325F) for 4 hours. Remove from oven. Sprinkle with powdered sugar and roll as you would a jelly roll. Sprinkle outside with a little more powdered sugar. Slice thin and serve.

## *Oatmeal Coconut Breakfast Bars*

1 cup quick oats
1 ½ cups apple juice
1 ½ cups all ~ purpose flour
½ cup toasted wheat germ
¾ cup shredded coconut, divided
2 tsp baking powder
½ tsp baking soda
1 tsp salt
1 cup packed brown sugar
½ cup unsweet apple sauce
2 cups grated carrots
2 eggs, lightly beaten

1. Preheat oven to 350°F. Grease a 13 x 9 inch baking pan.
2. In a microwave safe bowl, combine oatmeal and apple juice. Cover and heat on high 2 minutes. Let stand 10 minutes.
3. Combine flour, wheat germ, ½ cup coconut, baking powder, baking soda and salt. In a separate bowl, combine brown sugar, applesauce, carrots and eggs. Fold into flour mixture. Add oatmeal mixture and stir until just blended.
4. Spoon into baking dish. Sprinkle with remaining ¼ cup coconut. Bake 50 to 60 minutes, until a toothpick inserted in the center comes out clean. Cool and cut into bars. Serves 18.

## *Pizza Bread*

*What you will need:*          Shredded cheese

Loaf of French bread           Olives

A jar of spaghetti sauce       Pepperoni

Cut bread in half, lengthwise. Place on baking sheet. Spread both slices with sauce. Add above toppings (or your favorite), in layers. Top with cheese. Bake 8 to 10 minutes in 350°F oven. Remove and let set a few minutes before slicing. * Individual pizzas: slice as directed; then into 2 inch slices; continue as above. * * Substitute English muffins for French bread; continue as above.

## *After Thought Cookies*

*What you'll need:*

Graham Crackers                Heavy Cream

Powdered sugar                 Vanilla extract

Mix 3 cups powdered sugar with a few drops vanilla extract and just enough cream to make a nice 'frosting' consistency. Add more powdered sugar or cream, as needed. We like to add a drop or two of food coloring, also. Separate frosting into a couple of small bowls, and make different colors. They'll think you're pretty cool!

## *Egg Ocean*

| | |
|---|---|
| 6 eggs | ¼ tsp. salt |
| 1 cup flour | 6 Tbsp butter |
| 1 cup milk | |

Melt 6 Tbsp. butter in a 9 x 13 inch baking dish in 400°F oven. Meanwhile, mix eggs, flour, milk and salt. Pour into dish. Do not stir. Bake 20 minutes; It swells and puffs as it cooks; quite cool to watch! Remove from oven. Immediately sprinkle with powdered sugar. Serve warm with lemon, pad of butter, and syrup.

## *P B J Rolls*

Refrigerator Biscuits     Peanut Butter     Jelly

Roll out biscuits; spread with peanut butter; top with jelly; roll up like a jelly roll; slice one inch thick; bake as directed on biscuit package. The second part is Spiritual Fitness (the soul). The very breathe of our existence; our inner 'heart'; the part of mankind that hears what the heart has to say. The soul is that piece of you and I that feels joy and sorrow; love and hurt; peace and discontent. It desires more and more, each day; never quite satisfied, or fulfilled.

## Overnight Breakfast Bars

*Ingredients:*

*Bars:*

1 ¼ cups all ~ purpose flour
1 ½ cups old fashioned oats
2 Tbsp flax meal (optional)
1 tsp baking powder
1 Tbsp baking soda
¼ tsp salt
2 tsp ground cinnamon
1 cup granulated sugar
½ cup packed brown sugar
2/3 cup butter, softened
2 eggs, lightly beaten
1 ½ cups plain yogurt
2 medium apples,
   peel; core; and chop

*Topping:*

1 cup chopped walnuts
½ cup packed brown sugar
1 tsp ground cinnamon

*Directions:*

1. Preheat oven to 350°F; Grease a 13 x 9 inch baking dish.

2. To prepare bars, combine flour, oats, flax meal, baking powder, baking soda, salt and cinnamon in a medium bowl; set aside. Combine granulated sugar, brown sugar and butter in a large bowl. Beat with a mixer at low speed until just blended. Increase speed to high and beat well. Blend in eggs and buttermilk. Decrease speed to low and gradually add flour mixture, beat until just blended and scraping sides of bowl. Fold in apples, pour into pan.

3. To prepare topping, combine walnuts, brown sugar and cinnamon, mix well. Sprinkle evenly over batter. Cover with plastic wrap and refrigerate overnight.

4. Uncover pan and let stand 30 minutes. Bake 45 minutes, or until a wooden toothpick inserted in center comes out clean. Serve Warm. Serves 18.

## *Chive ~ Ham Bake*

*Ingredients & Directions:*

½ cup chopped onion

1 Tbsp butter

1 can (5oz) chunk ham, drained

1 medium tomato, chopped

1 pkg refrigerator rolls, in ¼'s

1 cup shredded cheese

2 eggs

¼ cup milk

¼ tsp dill weed

¼ tsp salt

1/8 tsp pepper

3 Tbsp minced chives

In a skillet, sauté onion in butter until tender; Stir in ham and tomato; set aside. Arrange biscuit sections in a (shallow) 13 x 9 inch baking dish. Spread ham mixture over biscuits; sprinkle with cheese. In a bowl, beat the eggs, milk, dill, salt and pepper; pour over cheese. Sprinkle with chives. Bake uncovered, at 350° for 25 to 30 minutes or until a knife inserted in the center comes out clean.

Yield: 8 servings. Serve with fruit, biscuits and cottage cheese (if desired)

## No ~ Bake Cookies

2 eggs
1 cup sugar
¾ cup butter
1 tsp. vanilla
30 graham crackers, crumbled

2 ½ cup cups miniature marshmallows
1 ½ cups nuts, chopped
4 Tbsp. coconut
Powdered sugar

Beat eggs in saucepan; add sugar and butter and cook over low heat until thick. Set aside to cool. Add vanilla, graham crackers, marshmallows, nuts and coconut. Mix thoroughly. Put into 9 x 9 pan and chill two hours. Cut and roll in sugar.

## Angel Pie

1 12oz pkg. vanilla wafers, crushed
2 Tbsp melted butter
2 cup powdered sugar
½ cup very soft butter

3 eggs, well beaten
¾ cup slivered almonds
1 large can crushed pineapple, drained
½ pint whipping cream

Mix wafers and butter and press into 9 x 13 glass baking dish, reserving some crumbs for top. Mix sugar, butter, and eggs and pour over crumbs. Sprinkle almonds over mixture; then sprinkle drained pineapple over mixture. Spread whipped cream on top and then sprinkle with remaining crumbs.

# Chapter

# Fifteen

### *Let's talk a little more about Faith:*

Do you believe in a higher power? Do you believe faith (or lack of it) makes a difference in a person's life? No, you do have to agree with me on this issue. This is just a question for you to answer; to you. Now, don't try the 'I'm not sure' approach. Either you believe; or you do not. Maybe means you have not made a decision regarding Faith in your life. Yes, a decision; you only have to decide one time.

If you have never been introduced to Faith; call me right this minute! Or, pick up your local telephone book's yellow pages and look under churches. Be careful; let your heart do the walking; your fingers will stop at the church you are to call. Faith is not about religion; it is about believing in Christ Jesus.

Believe me: Heavenly Father knows what you need. He will guide you. If you have been introduced to Faith; what is your stand on it? You've got to stand for something; or you'll fall for anything.

Faith is: Believing in some one or thing you can not touch, hear, or see. Yet, once you have been introduced to it, you may see that it was with you all along. Most of us believe a higher power does exist.

Sometimes, it just takes a while to figure it out. When our lives are going well, we become distracted. Though our Faith is with us, we do not act upon it. We put it on the 'back burner', and wait for a 'rainy day' to notice its presence, again. Does your Faith sustain you in difficult times? Sure it does. When we get into situations, we say 'Oh, my God'; or, 'Thank God'.

We swim across the water, believing our body will not fail. Do you drive a car; ride a train; take a taxi; or a bus? Are you not acting on Faith? Now, ask yourself, again: "Do I really have Faith?" Do I truly believe in a higher power? There are no grey lines to Faith. Answer yes or no. Now, you have made a decision. See how easy that was?

Now, back to my question: Does it make a difference whether or not you have Faith? I believe it does. And, if I am wrong: I've lived a Faith ~ filled life and have good vibes. In spite of it all (or because of) my life has been tough. And, it's been pretty easy. My perception vs. reality debate is never ending. Believing in a higher power does not guarantee us a sweet ride through life. It means we can trust our lives will go through ordeals we need to learn from, to get to the other side. Not a rose garden, baby.

No, there was never a promise of absolute peace on earth; that comes later. When we decide to believe, we decide, also to accept what ever comes our way with joy. No, really! Accept all things with joy:

knowing you will learn from the experience. This will require an effort on your part. What; work? Yes; if we never had to work at things; we would be as spoiled children who do not lift a finger. God loves us; He will not spoil us.

This work is called exercise. Not the physical kind, necessarily; an exercise of Faith. We may experience times of physical work necessary to full God's plan. Faith without work is dead. Maybe I should have said this earlier. Would it have made a difference? If life gives you lemons; make lemonade.

You decide how sweet it is. Just because a situation appears dark and dreary does not mean it has to be so. Ask what you can do to achieve the goal ahead. Do not go off half ~ cocked trying to 'fix things' on your own, if you have asked for greater interference. Oh, no; God does not need our help. He wants us to do our part in every situation: just, stay out of his way, okay? This makes it sweeter.

When my mother was hospitalized last fall (Emphysema) we knew she may not return home. Her health had withered over the past few years, and her body was headed down the exit aisle. I had two choices. One: Be sorrowful because I did not want her to leave me. Or, two: Be joyful; because she had lived a good life and was ready to go home.

Mom had Faith she was in good hands. She trusted me to care for her and follow her last wishes. Through this experience, I had new lessons in patience, understanding, tolerance, and compassion. Just when I thought I had been tested to the end, Heavenly Father tested me past my known strength. I learned Endurance.

# Chapter

# Sixteen

## *Endurance*

Endurance, my friend, is found through that strength we carry to the end. What ever we are going through, there is an end. Nothing lasts forever, here on earth. So, why do we complicate things? We live and learn, I suppose. Wouldn't it be nice if we could learn things the first time around, instead of reinventing the wheel? Nah; it would be way too easy.

When we believe there is an end to all things, our mind is less apt to wander to uncharted territory. In the midst of a catastrophe is the most common time to exercise our Faith. In those times, we are willing to work; to exercise our Faith. It's easy: Our Faith is there to sustain us. It's that one thing on which we can always rely. From birth, we have had it. It took us years to embrace it. Now, we find we no longer need to go on those roller coaster rides. Yippee! That's right; as we embrace our Faith, we are strengthened to endure to the end.

So, what happens when we do not have Faith? Remember the roller coaster rides? That's right. With out Faith, our soul is floating along, trapped in the body have been given. The mind can not fully rest.

Though some go through this life (seemingly) with out care; most are constantly searching for some thing. What, they do not know; some thing stronger and wiser than themselves. Their path is uncertain. They know not of an end.

The difference between the Faithful and those lacking in Faith is their understanding of the strength of a higher power. We do not have strength of our own; only that strength that is given to us. Our Faith, like our muscles, must be put to work to gain strength. If we do not 'work' on our Faith, we will lose our capacity to grow. With out that capacity, we would become stagnant. Our minds are an awesome wonder. However, they can get us in trouble real quick!

Our faith is tested through out our lives. As we make our way through trials, we grow and mature. We find strength to carry on, and endurance. Have you ever felt like you had more weight on your shoulders than you could handle? How did you get through the ordeal? The most important thing to remember, here, is that you did indeed get trough it. It may have consumed your every thought ~ for a time ~

However, you did get past that moment in your life. Trials are tests to help us gain strength. If we view them as a burden, our bodies may become weak. This lends way to colds, allergies, and anxiety.

Take a moment to reflect on the numerous trials you have been through since childhood. Do you recall how you felt during each of those times? Do you remember the details of every trial? No, probably not. Our minds have a unique way of sorting out good from bad; happy from sad; and important from let ~ it ~ go matters.

Though we may recall bits and pieces of an incident, our minds have already agreed with our spirits on which details should remain visible. Once in a while a negative point slips through; like when we are angry; tired; or insecure.

Negative energy promotes negative energy. If you want positive energy; it's up to you to take the bull by the horns and remove the negative from your mind. Take control of your thought process. Yes, you can. It's your line of thoughts, here: what direction do you want to go in?

Are you like a fast car; spinning out of control? Do you enjoy feeling so out of control? If not, do some thing to get a grip, man. Just put on the breaks; hold the wheel steady; and take a deep breathe. Believe me: it will come to a stop.

Race drivers understand the importance of a clean track. At high speeds, the smallest pebble can be dangerous. To ensure safety and a good race, the track is swept clean just a few moments prior to the race. Otherwise, the driver could be in danger of going into a tailspin; spinning out of control; Creating danger for all those on the track.

As we become anxious our minds race. Faith is like a strong wall with railings to grab along the way. Holding on to our faith helps slow us down. A slower pace allows us to regroup; and take a deep breath.

Positive energies can then reassess the situations at hand. The chaos that once encircled our thoughts is released. Though we may not be in control of every aspect of a situation, we are able to control our reactions. When we realize our level of responsibility, our life's positive energy becomes easier to sustain.

Without faith, we are more likely to allow our minds to race. Because we have nothing to grip onto to, it goes into a tailspin. The tongue is clever: it knows when the mind is out of control. An out of control mind gives the tongue permission to be out of control. Your mouth opens; words fly out; and the world around you goes into a tailspin. No one is safe from the danger. The daggers are released at will; the tongue has no mercy.

Now, this might be an interesting video game to play; but, c'mon, now. This is not just a game; it's your life we're talking about. You only get one round. There is no on and off button. The road you're heading down may pretend to be your friend; so be aware of the dangers.

# Chapter

# Seventeen

## Building a Positive Well Being

. If you have no faith, you are simply on your own. Well, that's the feeling you have, anyway. Truth is: we are never truly alone. If you have not determined where your strength comes from; you may be in deep danger. There are two powers that be: Higher Power (Heavenly Father; God; Allah); and the other power (Lucifer; Satan; the devil).

If Heavenly Father is not your source of strength then you may be allowing the other power to control you. Believe me; he will lie his way into your soul; your mind. What ever it takes to get you on his track Doubt; fear; insecurities; weakness; idle time on your hands: those things are the devil's playground. He'll even let you believe you've done the right thing. Oh, he is a clever one.

People of faith are not exempt from harassments from this evil one. The truth is: the stronger your faith; the more apt you are to be tested. Lucifer made several attempts to tempt Jesus. Jesus warned Lucifer not to tempt God. When we stand strong in our faith; holding to its strong arm, we have the power to resist temptations. We have the power to tell the adversary to leave us. This power also allows us to command him to stay away from our families; and our surroundings. Don't believe me? Try it ~~ it works!

Yes, faith is a marvelous gift. When tempted by negative actions; lift your heart upward; let your higher power be your strength. Draw near to it ~ and it will draw nearer to you. Just as frowning requires greater energy than a smile; faith releases the burden of doubt from your mind. Your soul is uplifted; positive energy renewed; and your face value is greatly increased.

By increasing your own face value; others notice the positive change in your demeanor. When surrounded by positive demeanor ~ life can not fail you. Allow your self the opportunity to build a positive well being. The joy you will feel in your heart will progress to your mind; and into your soul. Words are thoughts that are written on your heart. When we are unkind to one another, the negative words hurt the spirit.

The spirit warns the heart, who keeps note of the event. When the heart's filing cabinet gets full of pain and sorrow, it breaks. Some times the heart reacts with a physical explosion; a heart attack. Sadness to the heart is tough to recover from. One harsh word or unkind thing can wash away a ton of good.

Be kind to one another. We need to ~ for our own sake. Just an ounce of prevention is worth a pound a cure. In the same manner, one kind word can go a long, long way. A smile can wipe away the tears; a hug lifts the burden of loneliness; a handshake says 'Hello, it's nice to know you'. These simple gestures have such great value. When faith is the cornerstone of our lives, mountains that once stood in our way may crumble to the ground with a light touch.

Just as the Sun and Moon go round and round; so goes our lives. The Earth moves in the opposite direction of the Sun & Moon; revolving as friends; sharing each others values. Our circles of friends ~ like these planets are in the shape of a ball.

Although they may follow different paths, we know we can count on our friends to keep us on track: headed in the right direction. Such strength we gain from one another, sharing values and faith along life's way.

They say the friends we keep are a reflection of our true inner self. When we choose our friends through the pathways of our heart, we allow them to glow; as we become a reflection of their inner beauty. Our mind enjoys the benefit of the relationship; allowing our inner being to reflect through them. A true friend is the mirror in life that helps you see yourself more clearly.

Through the years, acquaintances come and go. We place distance and ideas between us. Somewhere along the way we lose touch. A true friend remembers the days gone by; always welcoming our presence. Though our lives have changed; we should not neglect our true friends.

### *Passing of the Friendship Ball*

*A ball is a circle, no beginning, no end*
*It keeps us together like our circle of friends and family*
*But the treasure inside for you to see*
*Is the treasure of friendship you've granted Me*
*Today I pass the friendship ball to you: Keep the Ball rolling*
*Here it goes; Pass it on to someone who is a friend to you*
*(Tell them to throw it back to someone who means something to them)*

'Rescue" a friendship over a cup of hot tea. It's amazing what a hot cup of Friendship Tea will do to the atmosphere. This ice ~ breaker is made to be shared.

### *Friendship Tea*

1 jar (18 ounces) Tang or store brand equivalent
1 cup instant iced tea
2 cups granulated sugar
1 package powdered lemonade mix
1 ½ teaspoon ground cinnamon
¾ teaspoon ground cloves

*To Store:* Mix; then divide into covered jars
(Or other containers to share)
*For hot tea:* mix 2 to 3 Tablespoon to 1 cup of hot water
*For iced tea:* substitute cold water and pour over ice.

# Chapter

# Eighteen

## *And, Life:*

Ah, yes! The existence we have been blessed with. Life is about living; learning; growing; achieving greater knowledge and understanding. Of what, you ask? Gaining an understanding of: Who we are; Where we came from; Why we are here; When we will leave this place; and What lies ahead.

Does it really matter, you ask? Let me ask this of you "When you travel, should you take a map?" Of course you should. If it didn't matter from whence we came, or where we are headed, we wouldn't need a mind to make decisions along the way.

Some say this place we call Earth will be destroyed; that a separation of heaven and hell will take its place. Some say we are already in a hell. Others, still, say there is no Heaven; and Hell does not exist (that we just came to life from the Earth).

I shall not deliberate these words with you. Each person is entitled to their own belief. Did we reincarnate? Did we come from the Spirit world, as the Bible indicates? Did we 'Spring up' from the Earth? One day, we may know: to day is not the day.

Let's say, for a moment, that the Bible is correct. Let's talk about this with an open mind, and an open heart. I will also note that I am not a scholar. No, I have not attended what the world views as 'formal seminary' classes. However, I did attend seminary classes at my church for four years. This level of learning shall be sufficient for the time.

Bible Courses are always a great source for knowledge, so long as they are taught from the least translated material. So many translations leave out words pertinent to the content. Information is available through many churches; libraries; and the internet on Bible Study Courses. Search; Ponder; and Pray before sending monies to any group or organization, regardless of their offerings.

Unfortunately, there are many who lie in wait to deceive. They present themselves as individuals; groups; even churches. It may take time to sort out the reputable groups. If you get a bad vibe ~ drop it like a hot potato and run! Good things will not hurt the soul; foul things are sugar ~ coated. When in doubt; get on your knees and pray about it.

So, to live a healthy physical life we first need to gain knowledge of the foods we are eating; water we drink; and the air that we breathe; correct? Now, we know this list could take up an entire book on its own, so we will keep it at food, water & air, okay?

Water was much purer 'way back when'. People actually drank it straight out of the water bed. No one worried about too much lead or contaminants. When necessary, they took a bath in the 'ol swimmin' hole, too. The same one their horses and cattle drank from. When was the last time you took a swim in a 'swimmin' hole'? Is there one around that has not been contaminated? If so, point me in its direction!

Many cities have public swimming pools. Open during the warmest months of the year, city pools must be treated with chlorine for purification. Do you know what happens to chlorine when you add heat? The heat gives it strength. Do you want extra strength chlorine on your skin? No thank you.

Now, the water plant supplying the city pool also supplies the homes within the city limits. (Same chlorine content; just no super charge) Either way, chlorine is in our water. The Food & Drug Associations and Environmental Protection Agency approve these chlorine levels for our consumption. Do you?

Well water is still the best, in most areas. Most rural areas still allow dwelling wells for new homes. Is it 100 % safe? No, not really. The trouble with well water is the minerals it contains. We won't go into the long list.

There are several ways to filter well water. The most important thing to address, here, is the dwelling of the well. When putting in a new well, make sure you dwell deep enough to avoid the 'bad water' on top; Get a nice, clean stream going and use a good pump.

Finally, we found ways to filter our water and provide it the public in an acceptable fashion. By placing it in bottles of all shapes and sizes, water has made its way to the grocers' cold cases. Bottled water now takes precedence to soft drinks. We buy pints; 1 liter; 2 liter; half gallons; and single or multiple gallons. This refreshing beverage and its healthy attributes are a hot item.

Now that we have caught on to the 'bottled water' craze; let's not forget to recycle the containers. At least we can find a trash container, so our land is not cluttered with empty plastic bottles. Plastic is a difficult product for the Earth to digest. It's not any healthier for Mother Earth than for your own body (and you know you can't digest it!).

Plastic is found in most man made products. Even our automobiles have gone from the steel production to this plastic stuff. Now, before there were automobiles, man actually walked or rode a horse. Most families had a buck board wagon they used for the trips into town; but, that was not a daily affair.

No, town trips were limited to once a week, at the most. The farther you lived out side of town, the fewer trips you made. Sunday was the exception: every body went to church. And, they didn't run clear across town two or three times a day just for a cup of coffee.

When did we get the idea walking was such a bad thing? Do you walk? It's okay; either way, you know I won't tell. If they'd allow my horse on the highway, I'd ride it to town. If you've been a horse, you know the work out you get. It takes energy to control even the best of such a critter. Now, I don't mind progress. I just think it paves the way to laziness and health problems. And, to keep our bodies fit, we know that exercise, food intake, and weight management are essential areas of focus.

How can we maintain a healthy physique if we never walk? Yes, it is possible. Many are not able to move about so freely. Though we should never use this as an excuse; some do. In the event your body is incapable of walking, we have a selection of routines that may work for you. Our exercises were designed with your limitations in mind.

Many fitness clubs are available to those with out restrictions. Too often outsiders lack understanding of physical limitations. Fitness programs are generally designed by thin, mobile, and well ~ fit individuals. That doesn't work for me; I don't expect it to work for you.

Careful consideration has been given to your disabilities. Do the best you can; at your own pace. No one else matters!

Move at your own pace; stretching your arms as only you can; and lifting your legs to a level that works best for you. The movement suggestions are just that: suggestions. This is what works best ~~ if you are able to achieve it. If not: do what you can, and don't worry about the rest! Just don't measure your best to some one else's; we are unique.

# Chapter

# Nineteen

## *Humans really are insecure creatures*

We ask opinions of others in every aspect of our lives. When it comes to health, we need to take control. Asking opinions is a good idea, for the most part. However, many people seek advice from several people for the same decision.

Though friends and family mean well, they do not always give the most honest response. They may be afraid of hurting your feelings; insecure in the own ideas; or even afraid of pushing your (negative) buttons. Maybe they know you too well. Know that no one can or will take care of you better than you will.

Our physical and mental abilities may be limited: that does not make us our own worst enemy. Each of has limits; we need to respect those limits of our self and of others. Have you ever wished you could do more or be more adequate? Most of us have. In doing so, we lose focus on God's plan for our life. Persons with disabilities have such a special place in this world. They are like angels with a body. Their demeanor is calm; at peace.

With so much love to give; and asking so little in return; their disabilities never get in the way of their life. A disabled person understands the values within each and every day. Yes, the values. Life gets so chaotic we often lose sight of its values.

What's so great about a new day? Everything! Are you kidding: each day is one more opportunity to lend a hand; share a smile; teach some one a new trick; or learn some thing new; and, that's just the tip of the iceberg: There's a world of opportunity out there.

*No matter how good things are*
*There's always something you need to be praying for*
*No matter how bad things are*
*There's always something to be thankful for*

Our friends and family provide the best sounding boards. When we're happy, they smile; our sadness shows in their eyes; heart ache bring tears, as they do their best to console us.

The individuals in your circle of friends and family were specially placed in your life to benefit you all. They live the miracle of your life along side you; day by day. Respecting one another's views and lifestyles; passions and dislikes; you travel together along life's merry lane. Imagine your life with out your circle.

Once upon a time, when a person wished to correspond with another, a formal letter was written; placed in an envelope; then in the mail box (with proper postage); and sent to the person to whom it was addressed. The receiver would respond in kind; thus, the phrase 'drop me a line, some time' was noted.

In today's world, we seldom receive hand ~ written letters. Back then, people took the time to write legibly. And, the receiver could actually decipher the message. Writing was an art; a language of its own. Have we forgotten the art of communication?

Maybe your hands are tired; sore from daily chores; paperwork, etc.

The balls of the fingers are supplied with a rich amount of nerve endings. Moving the hands and fingers in circular motions helps to stimulate blood flow.

*Here's a simple exercise for those tired, achy hands.*

First: Put a dollop of your favorite lotion in the palm of your hand
Next: Begin to apply the lotion to both hands
Clasp hands together and continue; letting your fingers move freely between each hand. Stop for a moment; retaining your grasp. Gently squeeze hands together; then release.
Next: Add an extra dab of lotion. Now, pretend you are washing them. Excess lotion should be applied to arms and elbows.

Go ahead ~ do this exercise through out the day. Anytime you need a quick 'pick ~ me ~ up', your body will be happy to oblige!

The following true story demonstrates an act of Faith.

### **The Miracle**

*A little girl went into her room and pulled a glass jelly jar from its hiding place in the closet. She poured the change out on the floor and counted it carefully. Three times, even. The total had to be exact perfect. No chance here for mistakes. Carefully placing the coins back in the jar and twisting on the cap, she slipped out the back door and made her way 6 blocks to Rexall's Drug Store with the big, red Indian Chief sign above the door.*

*She waited patiently for the pharmacist to give her some attention, but he was too busy at this moment. Tess twisted her feet to make a scuffing noise; Nothing. She cleared her throat with the most disgusting sound she could muster. No good. Finally she took a quarter from her glass jar and banged it on the glass counter. That did it!*

*"And what do you want?" the pharmacist asked in an annoyed tone of voice. "I'm talking to my brother from Chicago whom I haven't seen in ages" he said with out waiting for her reply to his question.*

*"Well, I want to talk to you about my brother," Tess answered back in the same annoyed tone. "He's really, really sick .... And I want to buy a miracle."*

"I beg your pardon?" said the pharmacist.

"His name is Andrew and he has something bad growing inside his head and my Daddy says only a miracle can save him now. So how much does a miracle cost?"

"We don't sell miracles here, little girl. I'm sorry but I can't help you." The pharmacist said, softening a little.

"Listen, I have the money to pay for it. If it isn't enough, I will get the rest. Just tell me how much it costs."

The pharmacist's brother was a well dressed man. He stooped down and asked the little girl, "What kind of a miracle does your brother need?"

"I don't know," Tess replied with her eyes welling up. I just know he's really sick and Mommy says he needs an operation. But my Daddy can't pay for it, so I want to use my money."

"How much do you have?" asked the man from Chicago.

"One dollar and eleven cents," Tess answered barely audible.

"And it's all the money I have, but I can get more if I need to."

"Well, what a coincidence" smiled the man "A dollar and eleven cents ~~ the exact price of a miracle for little brothers." He took her money in one hand, and with the other hand he grasped her mitten and said "Take me to where you live. I want to meet your parents. Let's see if I have the miracle you need."

That well dressed man was Dr. Carlton Armstrong: a surgeon specializing in neuro ~ surgery. The operation was completed free of charge and it wasn't long until Andrew was home again, and doing well.

Mom and Dad were happily talking about the chain of events that led to this place. "That surgery," her Mom whispered, "was a real miracle. I wonder how much it would have cost."

Tess smiled. She knew how much a miracle cost ... one dollar and eleven cents ...and the faith of a little child.

In our lives, we never know how many miracles we will need.
A miracle is not the suspension of natural law, but the operation of a higher law.

Now that you are rested ~~ maybe there's a friend you'd like to send a note to? When was the last time you actually looked at your address book? For most of us; once a year is more than enough. So it seems, anyway. Don't let procrastination get in your way ~ we only live once!

# Chapter

# Twenty

***About our Foods:***

The pioneers had the right idea, after all: grow your own food & vegetables; raise your own meat. They also made most of their own clothing and repaired their socks (save, save, save!). Where did they find time to complete all these tasks? Many of them had large families to care for. Where did they get the energy to accomplish all these things in a day's time? Oh, I forgot to mention how they carried water up from the river. (Whew!)

The foods we eat today have more additives than nutrients, and are packaged with more sodium than a person should have at one meal. Dieticians recommend that most of us should not consume more than 2400 calories per day. That might be reasonable for those who prepare meals at home, and take them to work or school. Can someone tell me how to keep within the limits while eating out? From what I've seen, it's not easy.

Aware of our concerns, the restaurant industry is finally making known the nutritional values of the foods they serve. Like most of the fast foods on the market, the foods I investigated were not what I consider healthy. The saturated fats; non saturated fats; sodium; sugars; carbohydrates; these are not on my healthy list. Are they on yours?

Yes, the pioneers knew good stuff when they saw it. A good meal meant no additives; except their own home grown spices.

On rare occasion, one might enjoy a between meal snack. When you're busy working, your concentration should be on the project at hand. Remember skipping lunch; because you were in the middle of a project, and didn't pay attention to the time? Your mind was so active your stomach didn't wish to interrupt it. Skipping breakfast is easy: we are in a hurry to get out the door.

But, don't worry: there's a McDonald's or a Starbuck's on the way; just grab a bite there, right? Its okay, most of us are guilty of that one! To make up for our lack of weekday nutrition, we find a good steak house on Friday night, or take the family to a nice buffet. Over filling our plates is a must; and we can't skip the ice cream and dessert section! Never mind leftovers; we'll grab a few munchies on the way home.

Oh, yeah ~ that's a real good idea. When the nine o'clock movie comes on, we'll pour some soda pop and set out the popped corn butter ~~ I mean, the buttered pop corn. Never mind the nutritional imbalance: After the week we've had, we deserve it.

A football game (especially the Super Bowl) is a grand excuse for more munchies than a person has a right to enjoy. And, no one dares to get between us and our munchies. Even our coworkers know not to cross that line. Of course, they will be happy to remind us of our growing waist line, now and again. Oh, they'll laugh, as though we should know it's just a joke. But, we know it isn't a joke ~~ it's the facts. (Ouch!)

Well, we are not going let a few extra calories spoil our fun; now, are we? (Of course not) The secret is to follow a few small rules.

*(Yes, we follow (most of) them, too!)*

Before you begin any new health regime take a moment to evaluate your current health status. Consult your physician. He can advise you which elements to count the intake of; either: calories; carbohydrates; sodium; or proteins.

The basic rules for making healthy changes include:

1. To help reduce the negative impact, start slow. Changing your daily eating habits may cause irritability.

2. Change one or two things a week, for the first month. Allow your mind to reset itself, as your body gets used to the changes. When we lose wait quickly; it will find its way back home (to our body) just as fast.

3. To drop the weight; and keep it off; we must learn new eating habits. That extra weight did not just 'suddenly' appear ~ give it time to go away; with out feeling guilty.

4. How is this guide different from the rest? We eliminated a big list of foods most people do not eat every day. Decision making is a whole lot easier.

## Counting Calories; Percents; Milligrams; and Grams

Personally, I am not if favor of counting calories. Anxiety runs wild, when I focus so many numbers before food reaches my taste buds. It seems the best way to keep track of the numbers is to carry around a pocket guide and a notebook; jotting down every morsel you munch on. My downfalls are carbohydrates and sodium.

The ultimate daily intake goal: Calories: about 1,200

How it should balance out:

Daily caloric intake (percent of value):
     Protein: 30 %    Carbohydrates: 45 %    Fat: 25 %
    * Food intake should supply a minimum of 30 grams daily fiber
On average, foods should be low in:
Sugar:   Minimum of 30 / Maximum 60 g
Sodium:  Minimum of 500 mg / Maximum 2,400 mg
Fat / Saturated Fat:
    *Women:* Max. 15 g per meal; 45 g day / Max.12 g Saturated Fat day
    *Men:* Max. 20 g per meal; 65 g day / Max.18 g Saturated Fat day
Cholesterol: Heart / High Risk Factors: 200 mg / General use: 300 mg
Fiber: Between 25 g and 35 g (recommended)

# Chapter

# Twenty One

*1*

**How Foods Count**

So, what foods can we indulge in while staying within the healthy guidelines? The following guidelines will help reduce the confusion. You may be surprised at the counts in foods you believed to be at the top of the 'healthier list'.

| **Noodles & Grains** | Serving | Calories | Protein | Carbs | Sodium |
|---|---|---|---|---|---|
| Egg Noodles | ½ cup | 106 | 4 g | 20 g | 6 mg |
| Elbow Macaroni | ½ cup | 87 | 4 g | 18.5 g | 2 mg |
| Spaghetti Noodles | ½ cup | 87 | 4 g | 18.5 g | 2 mg |
| Spinach Pasta | ½ cup | 91 | 3 g | 18 g | 10 mg |
| Brown Rice | ½ cup | 108 | 2.5 g | 22 g | 5 mg |
| Quinoa (keen ~ ah) | ½ cup | 106 | 6 g | 17 g | 6 mg |

| **Breads** | Serving | Calories | Protein | Carbs | Sodium |
|---|---|---|---|---|---|
| Whole Wheat | 1 slice | 73 | 3 g | 13.5 g | 155 mg |
| Rye | 1 slice | 83 | 3 g | 15 g | 211 mg |
| Bagel, plain | 3" round | 190 | 7 g | 37 g | 368 mg |
| English Muffin | 1 muffin | 127 | 5 g | 26 g | 218 mg |

*All counts based on foods that are: fresh; cooked (when applicable); No Salt Added*

| Meat & Poultry | Serving | Calories | Protein | Carbs | Sodium |
|---|---|---|---|---|---|
| Hamburger, 85% | 3 oz | 218 | 24 g | 0 g | 76 mg |
| Beef Round | 4 oz | 224 | 33 g | 0 g | 80 mg |
| T – Bone Steak | 4 oz | 237 | 29 g | 0 g | 80 mg |
| Pork Chops | 4 oz | 229 | 34 g | 0 g | 70 mg |
| Chicken Breast | 4 oz | 186 | 35 g | 0 g | 84 mg |
| Dark Meat | 4 oz | 232 | 31 g | 0 g | 105 mg |
| Turkey | 4 oz | 175 | 24 g | 0 g | 79 mg |

| Beans | Serving | Calories | Protein | Carbs | Sodium |
|---|---|---|---|---|---|
| Lentils | ½ cup | 115 | 9 g | 20 g | 2 mg |
| Kidney Beans | ½ cup | 112 | 8 g | 20 g | 2 mg |
| Lima Beans, baby | ½ cup | 115 | 7 g | 21 g | 3 mg |
| Garbanzos | ½ cup | 134 | 7 g | 22 g | 6 mg |

**\*\* Counts are for canned; condensed Soups & Stews \*\***

**\*\*\* t = trace amounts \*\*\***

| **Soups & Broth** | Serving | Calories | Protein | Carbs | Sodium |
|---|---|---|---|---|---|
| Beef Broth, cubes | 1 cup | 17 | 3 g | t | 782 mg |
| Chicken Broth, cubes | 1 cup | 39 | 5 g | 1 g | 776 mg |
| Chicken Noodle | 1 cup | 75 | 4 g | 9 g | 1106 mg |
| Cream of Celery | 1 cup | 64 | 3 g | 10 g | 838 mg |
| Cream of Potato | 1 cup | 73 | 2 g | 11 g | 1000 mg |
| Minestrone | 1 cup | 82 | 4 g | 11 g | 911 mg |
| Tomato | 1 cup | 85 | 2 g | 17 g | 695 mg |
| Vegetable | 1 cup | 122 | 3.5 g | 19 g | 1010 mg |
| Vegetable w/ Beef | 1 cup | 78 | 6 g | 10 g | 791 mg |

| **Vegetables** | Serving | Calories | Protein | Carbs | Sodium |
|---|---|---|---|---|---|
| Asparagus | ½ cup | 22 | 2 g | 4 g | 10 mg |
| Broccoli | 1 stalk | 78 | 8 g | 14 g | 10 mg |
| Celery | ½ cup | 14 | 1 g | 8 g | 51 mg |
| Carrots | ½ cup | 35 | 1 g | 8 g | 51 mg |
| Corn, yellow | ½ cup | 88 | 3 g | 20 g | 14 mg |
| Green beans | ½ cup | 14 | 1 g | 3 g | 1 mg |
| Lettuce, Iceberg | 1 cup | 7 | 1 g | 1 g | 5 mg |
| Lettuce, Romaine | 1 cup | 8 | 1 g | 1 g | 4 mg |
| Onions, yellow | ½ cup | 61 | 2 g | 14 g | 5 mg |
| Peas | ½ cup | 67 | 4 g | 13 g | 2 mg |
| Potatoes | 1 med | 156 | 3 g | 36 g | 379 mg |
| Sweet Potatoes | ½ cup | 103 | 2 g | 24 g | 10 mg |
| Tomatoes | 1 cup | 38 | 2 g | 8 g | 16 mg |
| Winter Squash | ½ cup | 40 | 1 g | 9 g | 1 mg |
| Zucchini | ½ cup | 14 | 1 g | 4 g | 3 mg |

| **Fruits, whole** | Serving | Calories | Protein | Carbs | Sodium |
|---|---|---|---|---|---|
| Apples | 1 fruit | 81 | t | 21 g | 28 mg |
| Banana | 1 fruit | 109 | t | 28 g | 1 mg |
| Blackberries | 1 cup | 75 | 1 g | 18 g | 0 mg |
| Cherries | 1 cup | 52 | 1 g | 125 g | 3 mg |
| Grapefruit | ½ fruit | 41 | 1 g | 10 g | 3 mg |
| Grapes | 1 cup | 114 | 1 g | 28 g | 3 mg |
| Peaches | 1 fruit | 68 | 1 g | 17 g | 3 mg |
| Pear | 1 fruit | 51 | 1 g | 13 g | 0 mg |
| Orange | 1 fruit | 64 | 1 g | 16 g | 1 mg |
| Raspberries | 1 cup | 60 | 1 g | 14 g | 0 mg |
| Watermelon | 1 cup | 49 | 1 g | 11 g | 3 mg |

| **Fruit Juices** | Serving | Calories | Protein | Carbs | Sodium |
|---|---|---|---|---|---|
| Apple Juice | 1 cup | 117 | t | 29 g | 7 mg |
| Orange Juice | 1 cup | 110 | 2 g | 25 g | 2 mg |
| Grape Juice | 1 cup | 154 | 1 g | 38 g | 8 mg |
| Grapefruit Juice | 1 cup | 101 | 1 g | 24 g | 2 mg |
| Prune Juice | ½ cup | 91 | 1 g | 22 g | 5 mg |
| Cranberry Juice | 1 cup | 45 | 0 g | 11 g | 7 mg |

Now, take a few minutes to check the items in your pantry. If you are serious about healthy eating, set aside food items high in sodium, calories, fats and sugars. Determine which foods you can live with out, and place them in a paper bag. The other items you can rotate within your menus. Take the bagged foods to a nearby shelter or food pantry. This will put a smile on your face; while helping the needy.

With this list of food counts in hand, grocery shopping will become much easier ~ and cheaper, too! If you like the idea of a healthier wallet, clip a few coupons from the newspaper. No, don't make your self too crazy, here. Actually, clipping coupons is a great way for your kids (or the neighbors') to learn how to save money. (Just a thought)

Before going to the market, make a list of the things you actually need. This may be a big change for your family. By changing our shopping habits, we are less apt to buy items we don't need. The cost of junk foods and soda add up real fast. So, cut those coupons; before you shop. After check out; look at your receipt. It should say how much money you saved. Then, go ahead: Smile! (It's okay to brag a bit, too!)

# Chapter

# Twenty Two

Along life's way don't forget to:

### *Add a Little Laughter*

Now, you know we need to do this one! Yes: Laughter. The very best way to enjoy the day is to fill it with the sounds of laughter. Go ahead; stretch your mouth from one side to the other. Part your lips; make a funny noise like: Ha, Ha, Ha! Don't worry about wrinkle lines, at a time like this! Laugh lines are much prettier than perturbed lines, anyway.

Before we can laugh; we must first turn our frown into a smile. The cheeks relax, and move upward. It's not a difficult task, really. In reality, a smile is much easier to present than a frown. That's right ~ easier. Frowning actually requires the use of more facial muscles than a smile does. It's a wonder more people don't catch on to this concept. I guess the simpler things are; the more complicated we make them out to be.

On a playground, the sounds of laughter fill the air. Children laugh; smile; play; and forget their everyday routines. Every one is their friend. A stranger is just some one they have not met before. Excitement abounds, as the swings fly up and up; merry go rounds go round and round. Life is awesome; no worries; no cares; just smiles and laughter. Oh, what a joy to be a kid!

How is it we forget this simple gift we have been given? Did we get so carried away with our routines that our smile got tired? Now, if you said yes ~~ you were not listening! A smile takes less energy than a frown. With grandkids around, it's hard to frown. So, don't be mad at me. I'm smiling at the moment! And, yes, we do get busy doing the ordinary things. We become creatures of routine. Too often, we just forget to enjoy life.

> *We don't forget to have fun; because we grow old ....*
> *..... We grow old; because we forget to have fun.*

At the age of 18, I moved to the San Francisco Bay Area. With my apartment just sixteen blocks from the ocean, I walked down to the beach often. The streets rolled up and down, much like a roller coaster. The walk down to the beach was great. The return walk was a bit challenging. After walking along the shore line for an hour or so, it seemed the trip home was twice the distance.

As the ocean waves splashed upon the shore, I felt a sense of peace. The crashing of the water on the rocks was like thunder to my ears. They moved with such calming strength. There presence was certain. Yet, my physical being was not moved by their flow. Seagulls landed nearby; then flew off into the sunset; unaware of my presence there.

The water was their playground. Just as children become oblivious to grown ups, this winged creation seemed oblivious to mankind. It's been said that seagulls have a fun life. Maybe they do. They swim; fish; watch those crazy people on the beach; flutter around in the sunshine; and lie around on the shore.

What a life. Maybe we could learn a few things from our feathered friends. I have never seen a seagull stand by and wait for another seagull to bring him his dinner, or pick up after him. No, they each have a job to do. No one gets to be a slacker. They exercise and eat well. What a concept. Have you ever seen a seagull that looks 'old'?

*Just in case you need a little encouragement:*

### The Canceler

A health nurse occasionally went to Lilly's school to give her breathing treatments. On one such visit, while they were in the teacher's lounge, a woman walked in; greeted Lilly; and left. "Who was that?" The nurse asked Lilly. "That was our school canceler" she replied. "Canceler?" "Yes, you know, canceler" Lilly said. "If a kid gets sick, they go in to see her, and she cancels it."

*(A true story ~~ hope it caught you smiling!)*

Ah, the wonder of a child. Remember when we laughed at cartoons; and told a silly April Fool's Day joke that you just had to laugh at (it was so dumb you either laughed or cried). How about rolling around on the grass with your arms around your waist because you laughed so hard that you fell down?

And, did you ever laugh so hard you thought you might have to change your clothes? Yes, laughter. The good old laugh ~ till ~ you ~ hurt kind of laughter. When was the last time you really did? Yeah, I know. Life got in the way, some where along the line, didn't it? Well, it's never too late to regroup. If your eyes opened this morning, and you can read this, now ~~ you can certainly still laugh!

Regardless how hectic your day has been; or who did what to sabotage it; or what kind of mood you are in; just try it one time. Honest ~~ it's amazing how wonderful it is to do this one little thing. And, if anyone else is in the vicinity, you might want to hold up a caution sign ~~ laughing can be very contagious.

The next time you are in a long line; try it. Start with a light chuckle; progressively getting a bit louder; and go into a good laugh. In a department store, or on an elevator, make sure others are around you, and try giggling like you just heard the funniest secret ever ~~ you will definitely draw a 'funny' crowd. Yes, we did try this: and, it did work!

Like I said before; I don't suggest you do anything that I won't do myself. Would you believe I am actually very conservative? Yes, it's true.

Being conservative has its advantages. When people view us as 'old fashioned'; conservative; dull; or maybe 'stickler's; they have a false sense of who we are. Glass walls are placed between us and them for fear we might enter their space. Their ideals are clouded by the versions they have created. Hence, they can not see the rose through the fogged glass. We must shatter their ideals and show them who we are.

All those years, we held back; watching from the sidelines as others stole the moment. At last, we are FREE! Be careful, now. Just a giggle or two, okay? Hold the really strong laughter for when you leave the frog in the boss' desk, and the guy across the room gets the rap. Then, take the elevator, and laugh out loud: Every one else with laugh with you. (Maybe that's not such a silly idea, after all)

### Kiss Me, You Fool

A guy is 85 years old and loves to fish.

He was sitting in his boat the other day when he heard a voice say, 'Pick me up.' He looked around and couldn't see any one. He thought he was dreaming when he heard the voice say, again, 'Pick me up.' He looked in the water and there, floating on the top, was a frog.

The man said, 'Are you talking to me?'

The frog said, 'Yes, I'm talking to you. Pick me up; then kiss me; and I'll turn into the most beautiful woman you have ever seen. I'll make sure that all your friends are envious and jealous because I will be your bride.'

The man looked at the frog for a short time, reached over; picked it up carefully, and put it in his front pocket. Then, the frog said, 'What, are you nuts? Didn't you hear what I said? I said kiss me, and I will be your beautiful bride."

He opened his pocket, looked at the frog and said, 'Nah, at my age I'd rather have a talking frog.'
*(Bet you laughed out loud ~ 'cause you know that there was funny!)*

# Chapter

# Twenty Three

## *About exercising:*

Exercising should feel good. If you over do it; you may pull a few muscles (that you didn't know you had). Our routines involve simple, everyday moves incorporated into a super ~ easy routine. And, you won't break the bank purchasing special equipment.

All of those special weights, mats, and equipment can be costly. Getting in shape shouldn't require a choice between buying food and a fitness routine. The two choices should go together. We don't like clutter; so we won't ask you to drag out a bunch of stuff.

Do you have just one dining room chair in your home? Yep, that's all you'll need: no kidding! By utilizing items already in your home, workouts can be done just about any time of the day. Multiple items just take up space in the closet, or under a bed. If you do own specialty items; feel free to use them. They might enhance the workout. Just don't over do it, okay?

*A few things to consider, before you begin:*

First: Ask you physician if it's okay, medically, for you to perform these exercises. Advice may be given regarding any limitations you may have. Be sure to follow the guidelines they set.

Second: Prior to doing each exercise. Review all steps. It's easier to complete the exercise when you are aware of all of the moves. Do not assume you know it already.

Third: Choose an 'Exercise Chair'. Using the same chair each time you exercise will keep your anxiety level down. Familiarity can be crucial for safety. Your mind will appreciate this little touch.

Fourth: Do not end a stretch without 'pulling through' it. Discomfort is caused by asking your muscles to do things they may not have done for a while. This may be counteracted by holding your body in that stretch for a moment; then stretching just a bit further.

Let your body be the guide. Your muscles will release; it just might take a moment or two.

If you feel cramping or your muscles pull with a sharp jab; Try not to tighten up. Pull your muscles just a hair farther, and let them relax. Do not drop out of the position quickly! This will hurt even worse. Just relax. Your body will release the discomfort. This process should just take a minute.

And, last, but not least: Be sure to adapt the level of exercise to your physical abilities. Whether you are young and strong; physically impaired; ambulatory; or in a wheelchair most of these exercises may be adapted to fit your personal physical levels. Disabilities vs. Abilities (You may want to stay away from the headstand)

*Okay; ready? Here we go!*

**Moves for the Body**

*Exercise Tip:* Balance Issues ~ standing close to your chair helps. Allow room to do the routine without hitting the chair with your head, arms, legs, etc.: try an arms length

### Stretch to the Sky

From a Standing Position: Stand behind your chair. Place one hand on back of chair. Raise your other hand upward toward the sky. Reach high. Allow your body to bend, slightly to the opposite side. At the farthest reach, count to five. Release slowly. Switch hands, and repeat moves; releasing slowly. Turn around, so your back is against the back of the chair. Raise both hands; clasp together as high above your head as possible; allow shoulders to roll backwards a bit.
Release slowly. Repeat the stretch & release moves.

From a Sitting Position: Hold Index finger and thumb together; raise them to your chin so it fits in the 'circle'. Raise elbow as high as you can; allowing neck to bend to opposite side, while shoulder rolls backward. At farthest reach, count to five; Release slowly. Switch arms; repeat moves as above, releasing slowly.

Next; Raise both hand behind your head, or neck; Clasp hands, if possible. Raise both elbows as high as you can; Count to five; Release slowly.

### *Reach out to Your Neighbor*

From a Standing Position: Stand with the back of your chair at one side. Place closest hand on back of chair. Stretch other arm outward, as if to touch your neighbor. Let your upper body bend, so you get a good stretch. Don't forget to wave! Release slowly. Switch sides, and repeat stretch & release moves. Again, don't forget to wave! Release slowly.

Alternating sides: Facing the chair, slowly stretch the upper body from one side to the other. Let the upright arm flow inward, as you bend. Touch the chair, if you feel off balance. Keep you back straight, not slouched; as you bend. Move slowly.

From a Sitting Position: Place one hand just below your chest. With the other hand, reach out to your side, as far as you can, and wiggle your fingers. Count to five. Switch hands, and repeat stretch and release moves. Move slowly.

Alternating Sides: From same starting position: Move from one side to another five times; moving slowly.

## Play Patty Cake with the Floor

From Standing Position: With your chair in front of you, reach down towards the floor. Make sure you have enough room to move, without hitting the chair. Touch both hands to the floor (or as far as you can) at the same time. Use your chair for stability, if needed.

From Sitting Position: Reach both hands downward, toward your feet. Stay within your comfort zone. Reach as far as you can; Count to five; Release slowly.

## Lung Forward and Kneel

From Standing Position: With feet positioned below your hips, lung forward with one leg, allowing your arms to lift up to shoulder height. Stretch your back forward as you count to five. Release slowly. Repeat lunging, alternating sides. Repeat five times per leg. Count to three between lunges. Do not skip this step!

From a Sitting Position: Hold sides of chair, near buttocks (or ends of chair arms). With out lifting your feet off the floor, use your thigh muscles to 'walk'. As you 'move' forward, other muscles may join in; it's okay. 'Walk' for ten to fifteen moves per leg.

## *Hindu Squat*

From a Standing Position: Feet slightly apart; arms at your side; back straight; chair within reach, in front of you. Slowly lower your buttocks, raising your arms out, in front of you to shoulder height. This should feel natural; not forced. Lower your body to a comfort point. Do not allow yourself to feel anxious. For support, touch the back of your chair with both hands. Using only one hand may throw you off balance. Count to five; then slowly return to the starting position. This exercise may be repeated up to ten times per session. Count to three between squats. Do not skip this step!

From Sitting Position: Sit upright; Grip sides of seat, near the front (chairs w/arms; hold arm ends. Extend feet to a comfortable sitting position. With knees together, lean as though pushing your chest to the wall in front of you; keep back straight. Release slowly. Repeat five times; releasing slowly.

## Headstand

From a Standing Position: From the squat position, place both hands on the floor, with hands inward, lifting buttocks. Elbows should bend outward, with wrists just outside the shoulder width. Lower the top of your head to the floor, facing behind you. Your elbows will naturally bend outwards. Practice this step a couple of times to make sure the spacing is comfortable. Raise your buttocks upward, allowing your knees to rest on your elbows. Continue upward until, smoothly, until the bottoms of your feet are facing the ceiling. Be careful not to over extend. Hold for a count of ten, if you can; Returning slowly to the starting position.

*Do not hold extended position! Injury to your neck/ back may occur*

Alternate Positioning: Begin this exercise facing a wall. Allow enough room to bend forward, leaving no more than a foot between your back and the wall. The wall will act as a support beam, if you over extend.     ** Warning applies **

From a Sitting Position: Bring your feet in, as close to the chair as possible. Reach your arms forward, stretching your back. Breathe in and out as your body relaxes. Hold onto your calves as you hold this position; Count to ten. Release very slowly; normal breathing is important. At the upright position, stretch both feet forward; Count to five.

### Chair Cycling; Walkin' Along; Heel Lifts; Raising the Ball; Teeter ~ Totter & Tipsy Toes

***Important Tip:*** *Continue repetitions as is comfortable. Do not over do this exercise! If you become winded, or feel discomfort: STOP! Hernias are not worth the effort!*

Begin with only five repetitions. Add up to five repetitions, two to three at a time, at your own pace. Allow three days between changes in number of repetitions for your body to adjust to the increase. Repeat this exercise for a maximum of ten sets, until your body is strong enough to do more. We recommend a *maximum* of twenty five sets.

### Chair Cycling

Normal Positioning: Sit at the edge of a chair; with your buttocks completely on the chair; and your legs free to bend. your hands on the edge of the chair, close to the back. Lean back just enough to allow your arms to support you. Bending one knee at a time, bring knee toward your upper body, and release; Alternate movement as though you are riding a bicycle. Use caution; and breathe normally. Do not allow your feet to touch the floor in between repetitions.

(Chair Cycling, con't.)

Alternate Position: Sit back (straight) in a chair; grip the edges, near your buttocks. (Or, grip the arm ends) With your legs taking turns; Use your thigh muscles to raise and lower your heels off the floor; with out lifting your toes. Follow above instructions. Use caution: if you feel a cramp in progress; STOP! It's not worth the pain.

### *Walkin' Along*

Standing Position: As though you were walking, lift one leg, then the other. Repeat this exercise up to ten times per leg; per set; as comfortable. Breathe normal. Count to three between sets. (1 ~ 5 sets)

Sitting Position: Sit back (straight) in a chair; grip the edges, near your buttocks. (Or, grip the arm ends) With your legs taking turns; Use both your buttocks and thigh muscles to raise and lower your heels off the floor; with out lifting your toes. Follow above instructions. Use caution: if you feel a cramp in progress; STOP!

## Heel Lifts

Standing Position: Place both hands on the back of your chair, for balance. Lift your heels, one at a time, to a comfortable height. Lift each heel five times per set. Count to three between sets. Continue as comfortable. (1 ~ 5 sets)

Sitting Position: Place both hands on the edge of your chair (end of arms). Lift your heels, one at a time, to a comfortable height. Lift each heel five times per set. Count to three between sets. Continue as comfortable.

## Raising the Ball

Standing Position: Hold your chair for balance. Lift the top (ball) of your foot to a comfortable height; and return to normal position (toes stay on floor): Alternate feet. Repeat this exercise up to five times per leg. Count to three between sets. (1 ~ 5 sets)

Sitting Position: Place both hands on the edge of your chair (end of arms). Lift the top of your feet, one at a time, to a comfortable height (heels stay down): Alternate feet. Repeat this exercise up to five times per leg. Count to three between sets. (1 ~ 5 sets)

## Teeter ~ Totter

Standing Position: Place both hands on back of chair. Roll back on your heels; then forward onto your toes; like a teeter ~ totter. Repeat five times per set. Count to three between sets. (1 ~ 5 sets)

Sitting Position: Place both hands on the edge of your chair (end of arms). Roll back on your heels; then forward onto your toes; like a teeter ~ totter. Repeat five times per set. Count to three between sets. (1 ~ 5 sets)

## Tipsy Toes

All Positions: Go ahead ~ take off your shoes! Raise your toes and wiggle them for a minute or two. You might want to count to ten. Count to three between sets. Repeat exercise up to five times. (1 ~ 5 sets)

### *Cat Stretch*

Release your body from the exercises: pretend you are a cat. Stretch our body out as best you can: Reach for the sky; stretch your legs toward the wall; Twist and stretch your back, hips and thighs; Round your back and release; Roll your neck and shoulders, as you go. Only do this one time.

Alternate Positioning: This exercise may be adapted to fit your physical abilities. Stretch to your own abilities. Do not push yourself! Only do this one time.

Let your body determine the best stretches. Yawn, as you go! Only do this stretch one time. You will be amazed at the relaxation and increase of energy this creates.

# Chapter

# Twenty Four

## Life Changes ~ *For the Soul*

*Exercise tip:* Balance issues ~ Silence is Golden
*Relaxation Tip:* A quiet room promotes tranquility


Though a quiet room may not be an easy option, it is essential to our well being that we set aside a few minutes, each day, to reclaim our personal space.

Women often soak in a warm bath; or pretend to read a book. Men close the office door, and hold a phone to their ear. Kids close their eyes, and pretend they're asleep.

A park bench; Back porch; garden; even a closet may be a good quiet place. Regardless of where it may be ~~ find yours.

How should you spend this precious, limited time? Read on!

## *Quiet Time Alone; With Me*

*1. Close your eyes*

Our mind is full of activity. When we close our eyes, our mind is able to focus on the matters at hand. Distractions of light, movement, color, and shapes are removed.

*2. Turn off the noise*

That's right! Take control of the remote; turn off your cell phone; and turn off the ringer to your landline telephone.

*3. Hang out the 'Do Not Disturb' sign* generally reserved for sentimental moments. Noise is 'clutter' to the mind and spirit. We clean up our messy rooms ~~ why not give our selves the same respect?

*4. Open the eyes of your heart*

Listen ~~ do you hear it? That tha ~ thump; tha ~ thump. Yes, that is your heart talking. Now that you are in a quiet place, you might actually hear it. Listen a few minutes longer, and you just might hear the many cries it has held onto. The joys; the sorrows; the desires: your heart needs your attention.

### 5. Listen to the call of your soul

Whether your life is full with joy; or discontent; your soul has a special need. That need is made known only through quiet, solitude. When we cleanse our minds from daily activities, we can listen more closely to the soul.

### 6. Respond with a Newness of Self

Information and findings are of no value, if we just put them on the shelf. Now you have prepared your physical body. You have listened to your soul.

As you practice healthy moves for your physical & spiritual health your body will react in ~ kind. Try it: you just might be amazed at the good changes!

So, what do I do next?

Your body and soul are ready to go to work for you, once again. They have regained their strength. What will you do with this new found strength? Maybe you could let go of those things that bogged you down, to begin with.

No, you do not have to forget about everything as though it never happened. Simply put: pick your fights. Maybe you have decisions to make; maybe bills that have to set unpaid; or, maybe you've just been too busy to spend time with those you care about most; even yourself.

*Yes, you CAN have it all!*

First: Breathe. Just breathe. Your mind is like a file cabinet. Once in a while, things get put in the wrong files, and you have to take a few minutes to reorganize. When we let it get out of hand, it becomes overwhelming to do the simplest tasks.

Now, write down everything that's on your 'mental list'. It doesn't need to be in any special order. Just write down everything that comes to mind; we all have to ~ do lists. Just write it all down; then prioritize. Don't try to complicate, here. You just relaxed; spent a few moments regrouping; and enjoyed a laugh or two: don't stop the ball from rolling, now. Get it all out in the open.

Now, when your list is complete, you can make choices. First off: do you wish to share the list with others? Or, would you rather destroy it? It's your list ~ you decide.

A few things to consider before your lists get too lengthy: Though it is much easier to jot down errors; rather than praise; we do tend to over look our own faults along the way. Out of all fairness, you may choose to reevaluate your notes before someone else gets a hold of them.

Question: As you created your list, did you happen to mention relationship repair? No, I'm not suggesting you need it; it does seem that we all have at least one relationship that could use a boost, now and again.

With that in mind, consider the ABC's of a Relationship. Are yours up to snuff? Are you willing to address them? Take a look; then decide if your relationships are 'just fine' or, if they could use a little attention. Maybe this list needs to be shared with others: You decide.

Here's an idea: Make a list of all of everyone close to you (friends; family; coworkers). Take a moment to reflect on relationships you have with each person on your list. Could any of them use improvement?

The following two pages address issues each of has in our relationships with other human beings. Because we are not yet perfected (not in this lifetime), we need to identify those issues and do our part to work on nurturing our bonds with those on our lists.

Whether they are casual acquaintances, or ones we hold dear, our efforts matter. Check out the Relationship ABC's ~ Give them your best shot!

# Chapter

# Twenty Five

## *Relationship ABC's*

A: Abandon Selfishness

B: Bestow Praise on One Another

C: Call Home if Running Late

D: Dream a Lot of Dreams Together

E: Enjoy Learning New Discoveries About One Another

F: Flowers Say A Lot

G: Grins Are Life Giving

H: Hands Are For Holding

I: Invest Your Time, Talent & Treasure On Your Marriage

J: Journey Together

K: Know How To Have Fun Together

L: Love Is A Decision

M: Make Time For Being Alone Together

N: Negativity Is Death Dealing In Any Relationship

O: Obliterate Jumping To Conclusions

P: Plan For Passion

Q: Quit Quarrelling ~ If it's Over 48 Hours Old; Let It Go!

R: Remember Those Special Days (Birthdays; Anniversaries)

S: Share Feelings On A Daily Basis

T: Take Lots Of Picture & Create Memories

U: Unity Creates Joy

V: Vacations Are Not Luxuries ~ Take Time To Recreate

W: Write Love Letters To One Another

X: Xmas Is A Time For Building Traditions; Not for Creating Tension

Y: Yearn For A Great Relationship; Not Just A Good One

Z: Zestfulness Breeds Excitement

*So, how did they measure up?*

Now, *make a second list.* Only this time prioritize the relationships. Don't get caught up on who is most important. Just make it basic: family first; then friends; then coworkers; the bank teller; grocery clerk; teachers. It's your list: you decide the order of importance. Maybe your thoughts are totally different from the examples. That's what makes us unique individuals: we have different thoughts.

*Remember this:* Each of us is entitled to our own personal thoughts. We have unique personalities, creating a wide range of thought patterns; circumstances; ideas; hopes; fears. Imagine what life might be like if we were all alike, in every way. BORING!

That's right: Boring!

Life is about adventure; learning; growing; becoming unique. Let's get back to that list, for a moment. How many names are on your list? Was your original list in order of importance? Would you like to add to the ABC's list?

As you can see, our lists grow and grow and grow and grow some more. Why is this? My guess is: every moment, our thoughts change. If we stayed in one thought pattern, we would become stagnant; and not grow. I know, I know; it might be nice to stop for a minute; right? Maybe it just sounds like a good idea. Would our lives be different? *(Maybe not so different, after all)*

Do you believe we are on this earth to stand still? Does your life ever stand still? Do you believe in a higher power? Or, are we a product of reincarnation? Though I can not read your mind, I believe we agree life does not stand still. So, why should our thoughts?

The next time you feel overwhelmed; anxious; depressed take a moment to find a quiet place to rest your mind and spirit. Let your body rest (not sleep), and not be weary. Cleanse you from within. Breathe. Lift your arms up high; stretch like a cat; and wave to your neighbor. Sit down; bow your head; close your eyes; cross you legs Indian style; and just breathe.

The rest of the world will go on without you, for a moment. They probably will not even notice you were gone. So, go ahead ~~ take five minutes for you! Yes, if you stay away too long, some one will surely notice. We take a minute to freshen up; make a call; get a cup of coffee. Why not take a moment to spend time with our self?

*It's one of the few things I can do for me; how about you?*

For everything we do; two choices always exist. Our choices begin anew, with each and every day. When we wake up in the morning, we can either go back to sleep; or get out of bed and join the crowd. Most of us get out of bed. Then, we either have breakfast in our pajamas; or get dressed and join the others (if any one else is around). As we go through our days, choices are many. No wonder we get so hungry; look at the work!

With all those choices, do we always make the right ones? Sometimes we can only hope to say we have done our best. Often, our choices are similar in effect, or out come. Does it really matter if we walk, or take the bus? What if I had held the door for the next guy; instead of being in such a hurry? When I pass the guy on the corner, should I give him a hand full of coins to maybe help his day?

Maybe we make good choices; maybe we don't. Maybe the good choices are the wrong choices; and the other choice was the right one. Who knows?

# Chapter

# Twenty Six

## Whole Body Wellness: Inside & Out

Okay; so our super human stamina helps to keep the household running. Who will keep us running? If we don't make our health a top priority; no one else will, either. We must take control of our daily lives ~ for the sake of our good health.

As we practice good health measures, the inside of our body gets plenty of attention. It is essential to remember to include the outside of the body, as well. Yes, the outside of our body requires just as much attention as the inside.

That doesn't mean hours at the spa (though it does sound inviting). We have some great tips that only take a few minutes for Gentle Facial Care (Cleanse; Tone; Moisturize; Exfoliate) and Acne Treatment. Then treat your body to a Mini Massage (Scalp; Hand; Feet). These easy steps will yield hours of appreciation (for your body; from you).

A warm bath does wonders to calm; relax; and revitalize your system. And, 'Yes'; we *do* have a few great tips for this, also!

### Gentle Facial Care:

Note: Facial cleansing involves the area from the forehead down to your collarbone; and just below the ears.

*Natural Facial Cleanser:* Almond or Sunflower Oil gently cleanses the skin; safe around eyes. Apply with a cotton ball (squeeze out excess). Use morning and night for best results.

*Toner: A splash of cold water! A cold wash cloth also does the trick.*

*Moisturize: Apply a light, oil ~ free moisturizer to moist skin; night and morning. Allow excess moisturizer to soak into skin.*

*Exfoliate: Moisten skin; apply Oatmeal Past (Recipe pg. 238); Rub with gentle, circular motions; Do not scrub; follow with sunscreen, if going outdoors.*

## Mini Massages:

*In just a few minutes your body can be quickly distressed.*

*Hands: Rub lotion into your knuckles and finger joints; then gently pull on the fingers, one at time. Massage the backs of your hands upward, towards the wrist (helps congestion).*

*Scalp: Beginning at the middle of your forehead: Gently rub the hairline; around ears; to the base of the skull. To release hands, allow fingers to flow across shoulders; outwards. Next: Brush your hair with a comfortable, stiff hair brush.*

*Feet: Wash your feet with a warm wash cloth. Apply a rich moisturizer. Gently rub your toes with your finger and thumb; continue for a minute or two. Follow with a soft pull of each toe; now, give your toes a minute to wiggle. (Feels great in the tub)*

**Now, to calm, relax & revitalize**

*A Warm Bath:*
Light a * candle; and stretch out in the tub. Place a rolled towel between your neck and the back of the tub for support, as you lean backwards. * Make sure the candle is on a safe, flat surface' to avoid falling or starting a fire.

*To Calm:*
Warm vanilla candles; rose petals; and a cup of hot chocolate

*For Relaxation:*
Add a cup of Epsom Salt; and a splash of lavender or chamomile oils; Hot Chamomile tea or a glass of red wine; and, of course: * candles

*To revitalize:*
Fruity bubble bath; a loofah or sponge; Fresh Linen Scent * candles; and a cold glass of Lemonade

# Chapter

# Twenty Seven

I'll leave you with one final story about choices; and how they can affect not only our lives; but the lives of others. Don't look for the punch line; 'cause there isn't one. Life is not a joke; it's a true story. So, read it, anyway.

**Two Choices**

*This is a true story. The child's name was not available; We'll call him 'Jake'.*

At a fundraising dinner for a school that serves children with learning disabilities, the father of one of the student delivered a speech that would never be forgotten by all who attended. After extolling the school and its dedicated staff, he offered a Question:

"When not interfered with by outside influences, every thing nature does is done with perfection. Yet, my son, Jake cannot learn things as other children do. He cannot understand things as other children do. Where is the natural order of things in my son?"

The audience was stilled by the query. The father continued. "I believe that when a child like Jake, who was mentally and physically disabled, comes into the world, an opportunity to realize true human nature presents itself, and it comes in the way other people treat that child."

Then, he told the following story:

Jake and I had walked past a park where some boys were playing baseball. Jake asked, "Do you think they'll let me play?" I knew that most of the boys would not want someone like Jake on their team, but as a father I also understood that if my son were allowed to play, it would give him a much ~ needed sense of belonging and some confidence to be accepted by others in spite of his handicaps.

I approached one of the boys on the field and asked (not expecting much) if Jake could play. The boy looked around for guidance and said, "We're losing by six runs and the game is in the eighth inning. I guess he can be on our team and we'll try to put him in to bat in the ninth inning.

Jake struggled over to the team's bench and, with a broad smile, put on a team shirt. I watched with a tear in my eye and warmth I my heart. The boys saw my joy at my son being accepted. In the bottom of the eighth inning, Jake's team scored a few runs but was still behind by three.

In the top of the ninth inning, Jake put on a glove and played in the right field. Even though no hits came his way, he was obviously ecstatic just to be in the game. And on the field; grinning from ear to ear as I waved to him from the stands. In the bottom of the ninth inning, Jake's team scored again.

Now, with two outs and the bases loaded, the potential winning run was on base and Jake was scheduled to be next at bat. At this juncture, do they let Jake bat and give away their chance to win the game?

Surprisingly, Jake was given the bat. Everyone knew that a hit was all but impossible because Jake didn't even know how to hold the bat properly, much less connect with the ball.

However, as Jake stepped up to the plate, the pitcher, recognizing that the other team was putting winning aside for this moment in Jake's life, moved in a few steps to lob the ball in softly so Jake could at least make contact.

The first pitch came and Jake swung clumsily and missed. The pitcher again took a few steps forward to toss the ball softly towards Jake. As the pitch came in, Jake swung at the ball and hit a slow ground ball right back to the pitcher. The game would now be over.

The pitcher picked up the soft grounder and could have easily thrown the ball to the first baseman. Jake would have been out and that would have been the end of the game.
Instead, the pitcher threw the ball right over the first baseman's head, out of reach of all the team mates.

Everyone from the stands and both teams started yelling, "Jake, run to first! Run to first!" Never in his life had Jake ever run that far, but he made it to first base. Jake scampered down the baseline, wide ~ eyed

and startled. Everyone yelled. "Run to second, run to second!"
Catching his breath, Jake awkwardly ran towards second, gleaming and struggling to make it to the base.

By the time Jake rounded towards second base, the right fielder had the ball: The smallest guy on their team; who now had his first chance to be the hero for his team.

He could have thrown the ball to the second baseman for the tag, but he understood the pitcher's intentions so he, too, intentionally threw the ball high and far over the third baseman's head. Jake ran toward third base deliriously as the runners ahead of him circled the bases toward home.

All were screaming. "Jake, Jake, Jake, all the WAY Jake". Jake reached third base because the opposing shortstop ran to help him by turning him in the right direction of third base, and shouted, "Run to third!"

As Jake rounded third, the boys from both teams, and the spectators, were on their feet screaming, "Jake, run home! Run home!" Jake ran to home, stepped on the plate, and was cheered as the hero who hit the grand slam and won the game for his team.

"That day", said the father softly with tear now rolling down his face, "the boys from both teams helped bring a piece of true love and humanity into this world."

Jake didn't make it to another summer. He died that winter, having never forgotten being a hero and making me so happy; and coming home and seeing his mother tearfully embrace her little hero of the day!

*And, now, a little footnote to this story:*

We all have opportunities every single day to help realize the 'natural order of things'. So many seemingly trivial interactions between two people present us with two choices: Will you make the right choices?

*May your day be a Jake Day!*

It's amazing how it all works together, isn't it? *Question is: Would you have made the same choice?*

*To help your day be the best it can be: Search; Ponder and Pray*

*Search* within; search the scriptures; search your 'energy' field.

*Ponder* the facts and information before you; the words of a spiritual counselor.

*Pray* for peace; guidance; strength; a cleansing of your soul; direction.

These are the things we must do to prepare our minds and our souls for this world.

So, relax; eat healthy; have a little fun; share a hot cup of Tea with a friend; get some exercise; rebuild a relationship with your higher power; find you; and enjoy life; with

*Simple Moves*

*For The*

*Body & Soul*

# The End

## *Go ahead; Quote me!*

*\* I have yet to hear a man ask advice on how to combine a marriage and a career \**

*\* If you want breakfast in bed; sleep in the kitchen \**

*\* A woman is like a tea bag
You don't know how strong she is
Until you put her in hot water \**

*\* Coffee; Chocolate; Men
Some Things Are Just
Better Rich \**

*\* Of course I don't look busy; I did it right the first time \**

*\* I have an attitude; and I know how to use it \**

*\* Do not start with me; you will not win \**

# About the Author:

Jana worked as an In Home Caregiver for over seven years. She has learned how to move forward through both personal and professional experiences. In 1990, a severe back injury: Options: back surgery; or spend the remainder of her lifetime in a wheelchair. She chose to have surgery.

The next eighteen years brought the use of wheelchairs; walkers; bed pans and In Home Care. In 2001, she had a second back surgery; and in 2003 was diagnosed with Rectal Cancer. Jana was blessed with instructions on personal fitness for her level of ability; which so many do not receive.

*Simple Moves For The Body & Soul*

*'Finding abilities*

*Through times of dis ~ ability'*

*This wonderful Whole Body Wellness guide is for individuals of all levels of ability. Jana shares with us a variety of elements to help cleanse and nurture our*

*Body; Mind; and Spirit*

*Topics include:*

*Health*

*Feel ~ Good Foods*

*Emotional Roller Coasters*

*Quick & Easy Recipes*

*Food Counts*

*Relationship ABC's*

*Exercise*

*Whole Body Wellness*

www.ingramcontent.com/pod-product-compliance
Lightning Source LLC
Chambersburg PA
CBHW032249150426
43195CB00008BA/379